QUALITY OF SLEEP, MOOD SWINGS, IMPULSIVITY AND EMPATHY IN RELATION TO WORK RELATED QUALITY OF LIFE AMONG DOCTORS

Supervisor:

PROF. SHALINI SINGH

Submitted By:

VARENYAM

ACKNOWLEDGEMENTS

The task of acknowledging the incalculable debt of appreciation which is owed to many is a very pleasing facet of thesis writing. It gives one immense pleasure in thanking those who were associated with me in completion of this work.

Firstly, I would like to place on record my deep sense of gratitude and love to **Dr. Shalini Singh** (Professor), Department of Psychology, M. D. University, Rohtak for her generous guidance, help and useful suggestions. I am short of words to thank ma'am for her support and understanding. Her encouragement to attempt a new approach is the trust that motivated me to carry this work forward. Her valuable advice, expert guidance, encouragement, constructive criticism, patience, motivation, enthusiasm, and immense knowledge provided me excellent working facilities throughout the course of this study. I have great respect and gratitude for ma'am. Thank you ma'am for always pushing me towards my goals and for being my source of guidance and knowledge.

I express my sincere gratitude to **Dr. Sonia Malik** (HOD, Department of Psychology, MDU, Rohtak) for providing facilities for this work. She is a woman with great vision and enthusiasm which has always inspired me. The discipline and values which she instilled in me will remain with me forever. She has always been so easy to talk to and discuss your queries, her empathy and understanding towards her students has always impressed me.

I am also thankful to all the teachers of **Department of Psychology, M.D. University, Rohtak**, for their co-operation, encouragement and valuable suggestions from time to time. Also, I express my sincere thanks to the non teaching staff of Department of Psychology, M.D. University, Rohtak, who provided me the material from time to time, needed for conducting the research.

I am deeply grateful to all the subjects who participated in the study and my friends, who acted as a confederate, without their help data collection would have not been possible.

I express deep thanks and heartfelt love and gratitude to my most caring and loving parents, **Dr. Arun Singh** and **Dr. Sangeeta Nehra**, for the encouragement, support and motivation that they showered in the completion of this project. My father has always stood by my side and his vision and unconditional support is one of the reasons I am a confidant and knowledgeable woman today. My mother has been my strongest supporter all along, her patience and inputs helped me a lot during my research. This altogether has actually helped me a lot to grow better and wiser. Her unending belief and confidence in me has helped me in achieving and retaining many things. My family has been strength during this study by making my everyday life easier. Their invaluable love, help, support and trust has given me the patience and courage to accomplish this work. I am also indebted to all other family members for their encouragement and timely advice.

I must also express my thanks to **Vijayanth Hooda,** my husband, my pillar in this journey for his never ending support. He's helped me a lot from time to time. He is my problem solver when I panic or am confused. His presence makes me feel positive and loved. He has always believed in me and helped me stay focused and encouraged.

My research colleagues have been an indelible part of my journey as well, especially my friend Arjun Sharma and my senior Dr. Ravi Rathee. Their guidance and support have been very important during the work on this title. My life has been touched and enriched by such amazing people, who believed in me even when I was not so confident, who heard me out, who encouraged me, guided me when I needed it, who made my journey easier and helped me achieve and see this day.

I am also thankful to the staff members of library of M. D. University, Rohtak who helped me directly or indirectly in fulfillment of this thesis work.

Thank you all and many others whom I have not mentioned here but without their support the present research would not have accomplished. Not only did the ones, in person helped me, I am also very thankful to God for being with me and watching over me. Hope his benevolence continues.

CONTENTS

LIST OF TABLES

LIST OF APPENDICES

Sr. No.	Title of Appendix
1.	Sleep Quality Scale (2006)
2.	Positive and Negative Affect Schedule (1988)
3.	Barratt Impulsiveness Scale
4.	Empathy Quotient
5.	Work-Related Quality of Life scale (2012)
6.	Paper Presentation

LIST OF ABBREVIATION

BPD	Borderline Personality Disorder
ADHD	Attention Deficit hyperactivity Disorder
QoWL	Quality of Working Life
ProQoL	Professional Quality of Life
HR-QoL	Health Related Quality of Life

CHAPTER – 1

INTRODUCTION

As the healthcare sector continues to concentrate on enhancing patient outcomes and greater satisfaction, doctors are working to develop their expertise as patient professionals. The most significant form of healthcare available to us today is physicians. In circumstances of clinical ambiguity and uncertainty, their everyday lives require them to take ultimate responsibility for challenging choices, building on their empirical experience and well defined clinical judgement. Doctors are a specialist subset of healthcare professionals who sometimes have to undergo heavy work at their workplace, often feel an unsafe kind of environment, very long time of work or pressurized working and overall, it leads to more level of stress and burnout.

They are a critical component of frontline health care. Doctors' well-being can directly relate to the quality of patient care. As per the International Labour Organization: "In order to prevent, diagnose, care for and treat patients with illness, illness and injury and to maintain physical and mental health, doctors as clinical scientists apply the principles and procedures of medicine." In the health care team, they supervise the execution of care and treatment plans by others and perform patient education and research.

Workers' health is potentially at risk from the job itself in each hospital department (e.g., stressors at work); ecological factors (e.g., toxic substances, ventilation inefficiency, radiation and bacteria); and the way timing of work (e.g., illness resulting from standing and sitting, shift work, and relatively long hours). When doctors face these threats and challenges, the standard of medical care would be affected.

For a healthcare institution to thrive, a doctor is the main resource. As critical healthcare gatekeepers and custodians, a doctor's position in the healthcare industry can be considered. It can, therefore, be mentioned that it means consulting a doctor to approach a healthcare institution and derive benefits directly. Increasingly, the healthcare industry is dependent on health workers i.e. doctors to treat well their patients. In the recent time i.e. 21st century, doctors are very much busy at their workplace and feel overburdened and lack needful resources. Shifting in their day-night timing on a frequently basis leads to disturbance in their sleep. Sleep is very essential for a body to restore its balance, mood and freshness. The way one tries to sleep and the previous day he had kind of sleep also effects mood and behavior of an individual including his/her attitude. It's hard to overemphasize the need for sleep. The lack of quality of sleep is connected to a variety of acute and chronic issues that challenge our everyday life. Sleep is a crucial component of human physiology, and sleep disorders can contribute to severe disruption of human functionality.

Now the question is, will we want him to perform his duty the next day if a doctor is operating late the night before and has not had enough sleep? These things are entirely contradictory to a doctor's virtues and the ethical moral code they pledge to uphold, which makes good sleep quality an important factor in a doctor's overall mental and physical health.

Quality of sleep

Simply put, sleep quality refers to how well you sleep. Adults should be able to fall asleep within a timespan of thirty minutes. A good quality of sleep is found to be effective when an individual is able to sleep properly with only one awakening and can drift back to sleep if they want so. The primary factors of quality sleep, according to the National Sleep Foundation (2019), include *"sleeping longer in bed (at least 85% of the time), falling asleep in 30 minutes or less, waking up no more than once each night, and being awake after falling asleep for 20 minutes or less."*

Sleep deprivation can cause physical and mental health issues, as well as injury, lost productivity, and an increased chance of death. People with behaviorally induced poor sleep syndrome are those who engage in voluntary, but unintended, chronic sleep deprivation. Sleep quality can vary. Hypersomnia or excessive sleepiness is another form of disorder associated with sleep. It involves feeling excessive sleepiness during the day that is present for at least three months almost daily. Long work hours, personal obligations and medical conditions can be other reasons for lack of sleep quality.

Fatigue, daytime sleepiness, clumsiness and increased appetite can lead to weight gain due to a sleep-restricted state (Taheri& Lin, 2004) and it also affects the brain and cognitive functioning (Alhola&Kantola, 2007). The amount of sleep needed for best health is seven to eight hours each night for most adults. When we get less sleep than that, it can eventually lead to a lot of health issues, as many people do. These are oblivion, inattention, low immunity, and even mood swings. Many busy individuals try to adjust their schedule to get as much done as possible, the quality of sleep becomes poorer and sleep is sacrificed. Older adults need as much sleep as younger adults; they typically sleep more easily than younger people and for shorter periods of time.

Several studies have looked into the relationship between sleep quality and how a person feels when they first wake up and throughout the day (Argyropoulos, Hicks, & Nash, 2003). The findings reveal that sleep quality is linked to waking ease, exhaustion, sensation of balance and coordination clarity, how one feels rested, restored, and refreshed, as well as waking mood and bodily feelings. Fatigue was associated with poorer quality of sleep during the day, while attentiveness was linked to higher sleep quality. External factors such as gender, scholastic accomplishment, academic background, health status, socio-economic status, and the individual's degree of stress, according to Saygili, Akinci, Arikan, and Dereli (2011), affect sleep quality. Mayda, Kasap, Yildirim, Yilmaz, Derdiyok and Ertan (2012) have also found that medical students may have sleep problems due to the fact that their training programme requires time and effort. Because of this issue, there may be various physical, social, psychological issues for students who can not sleep enough.

Stricker, Brown, Wetherell, and Drummond (2009) present empirical existing research that there is a brain area named as prefrontal cortex which is usually responsible for working memory and executive functioning including logical reasoning, it showed more activity in those subjects who are feeling sleepy as they tried to compensate for the negative effects of poor sleep quality.

The effects of the quality of sleep on physicians are underrated. Deprived sleep can make an individual drowsy and includes low mental efforts in a particular task, it also decreases self-confidence, there is a lack of emotional aspects and usually it leads to mood swings. A direct connection has been found between deprived sleep and mood swings.

Indicators of disturbed sleep

Sleep is a kind of biological state of body where a person wants to relax physically as well as psychologically and responses of an individual diminishes as one goes deeper into sleep. A tired response from a body while feeling sleep shows a disturbance in sleep. When we are more deprived of sleep, our cognitive functioning starts losing control and one can easily recognize from his/her body response about the severity level of sleep. Sleep deprivation can also be measured with the help of biological equipment's i.e. EEG, GSR etc. Responses of sleeper are then recorded and tested to identify the disturbance and severity of sleep.

Disturbance factors

The surrounding environment of an individual i.e. sleeper can be explained in the form of physical elements that contribute to his/ her comfort or discomfort. As a result it is a necessary part to record the level of physical stimulus i.e. outer temperature, humidity and light to find out the contributors of disturbed sleep. One must focus upon environmental as well as personal factors.

Sleep disturbances can be difficult to diagnose since they are frequently caused by a mix of physical variables encountered in daily living. However, because they affect the real exposure of the sleeper, it is vital to understand their respective levels as well as the amplitude of their probable variations. Despite the many evidence present in this time, there are only few publications related to the impact of environmental elements on human sleep.

Responsiveness of the sleeper

The ability of the sleeper to detect sensations via special sensory organs and send their signals to the associated parts of the central nervous system is crucial to his or her response. Detection thresholds, on the other hand, might be significantly altered while sleeping. If one wants to observe physical properties in a detailed way then one must see all possible reactions of environment and has to make a hierarchical order from mild to severe form of environmental stressors which causes sleep deprivation. As a result, a physical element capable of rapidly changing its properties, such as noise, can only produce very quick responses a few seconds after stimulation begins (Muzet & Naitoh, 1977; Muzet, 1989). A slowly changing physical component, like as ambient temperature, creates changes that are considerably more difficult to identify since they occur more gradually, despite the fact that their amplitude and final effect on the pattern of sleep might be significant.

The measure of responsiveness during sleep

Some of the immediate impacts of unsettling events can be noticed by the sleeper's easy visual inspection, such as extension of the falling fast asleep latency, rapid awareness, body movements, or postural alteration. EEGs, bodily changes, heart beat and respiration rate, vasomotor reactions, and sleeper pulse rate were all recorded polygraphically. However, polygraph provide more information on the evolution of the sleeping process, but most often remain reserved for the sleeping laboratory. Due to the disturbing factor, these recordings allow the detection of immediate effects.

The following are examples of immediate effects:

➤ Electroencephalogram alterations, which indicate mild to profound changes in sleep formation, ranging from distinct alertness to sleep stage transition or waking;

➤ Alterations in heart and respiratory rates and amplitudes, which are frequently linked to vasomotor and blood pressure changes);

➤ Motor responses, which range from minor limb movement to global postural change.

Factors influencing sleeper responsiveness

The research related to this concept is extremely difficult due to the numerous aspects that must be considered. The type of sleep, personal circumstances, and other situational factors should all be considered when determining the stimulus's properties.

Stages of sleep and deepness of sleep

The assessment of the awakening threshold is typically used in the traditional assessment of responsiveness. The initial measurement of sleep depth was dependent on the awakening threshold, utilising varied intensities and delivered at different times of the night due to noise stimulation (Kohlschütter, 1862). A significant increase was seen with awakening threshold usually at the end of first hour of sleep. Michelson discovered a curve in 1897 that showed similar fluctuations but with multiple undulations in the awakening threshold. Regardless of a stimulus utilized, all analyses revealed the presence of a deep sleep stage two hours afterwards falling asleep, followed by a shallower sleep stage the following hours. The abundance of certain distinct EEG activity and, as a result, the sleep stage might be employed as indications of the change in sleeper reactivity exposed to external stimuli in the earliest research using an electroencephalogram (Blake & Gerard, 1937; Blake et al., 1939). These research have led to the suggestion that EEG could be utilized as a sleep depth indicator.

Individual factors

Among the most often evaluated individual characteristics are age, gender, and psychological conditions.. When employing sound stimuli, there is a contrast in EEG responses among children and adults, with the former having lower brain wave stimulus responsiveness than the latter. This result, on the other hand, contrasts with such a cardiovascular sensibility that is nearly identical across age groups (Muzet et al., 1981).

The substantial disparities found between people are explained in part by the individual's attitude more towards a predicted wakeup owing to an identifiable trigger. Using self-assessment of noise responsiveness as a set of criteria, there was no massive distinction in measured cardiovascular reactivity while at sleep among subjects who considered themselves to be highly susceptible to loud and subjects who did not consider themselves to be highly sensitive to noise, despite a clear modification in reactivity between both the two groups throughout their wakes (Di Nisi et al., 1990).

Situation factors

There are numerous factors in the situation and some of them could have a modulatory effect on sleep reactivity. It is possible to manipulate some of these factors consciously. For prior sleep deprivation, this is the case. In this case, recovery sleep is characterized by a marked rise in waking thresholds after total sleep deprivation (Naitoh 1976; Williams et al., 1964).

The sleeper's response to noise can be modified by pharmacological sleep manipulation. But there is a dissociation between a reduced global disorder (awakening) and cardiovascular responses that are not modified after a sleeping medication intake (Muzet et al., 1983).

Mood Swings

A mood swing is a concept in which there is rapid change in mood having a particular reason for it. Severity of mood swings can also lead to formation of bipolar disorder. Mood swings are the kind of phenomena which can occur at any time and at any place, ranging from tiny to furious manic depression oscillation, so a continuum can be established from normal self-esteem difficulties to depressive disorder.

Mood swings might sometimes last for a long time. They can last a few hours (hyper rapid) or days (long) (ultrafine). When four consecutive days of hypomania as well as seven days of mania occur, clinicians think that a diagnosis of bipolar disorder is appropriate (Ghaemi,2007). Mood swings can last for days, even weeks, in such cases: these episodes may include a quick switch between depressive and euphoric feelings (Hockenbury, Don & Sandra, 2011).

Changes in a person's sleep patterns, energy level, self-esteem, focus, or drug or alcohol usage could all be symptoms of an impending mood illness. Mood swings can be caused by a variety of factors, including an unhealthy diet or lifestyle, substance misuse, or hormonal imbalance. Other important reasons of mood swings include diseases/disorders that interfere with the nervous system's function (besides bi-polar disorder and major depression). Attention Deficit- Hyperactivity Disorder (ADHD), epilepsy, and autism are three instances.

Causes of mood swings

It's not known exactly what causes mood swings. It is thought that the moods of a person may arise from chemical reactions in the brain. Thus, the result of chemical imbalances may be rapid mood changes. Sleep, diet, medication, and other lifestyle variables may also affect mood, and changes in these possibly will affect the steadiness of a person's mood.

Individuals who are going through a difficult time in their lives are more likely to have unexpected, unexplainable mood swings. Many teenagers, for example, may have frequent and erratic mood swings. These emotional shifts might be caused by challenges with identity, self-image, and acceptance. A individual who is already under lot of stress may also be more likely to have mood fluctuations. When a person is under a lot of stress, even a minor unpleasant occurrence might cause sudden mood shifts.

Mood swings can be caused by a variety of medical and psychiatric problems, including:

Bipolar disorder, borderline personality disorder, depression, schizophrenia, ADHD, and addiction are all mental health problems.

➢ Hormonal imbalances and their consequences
➢ Alzheimer's disease, brain tumours, meningitis, or other disorders affecting the central nervous system
➢ Thyroid conditions
➢ Lung or cardiovascular illnesses that impair the transport of nutrients as well as oxygen to the brain
➢ Anxiety, depression, and other forms of emotional discomfort

Mood swings are treatable but with proper care and precautions. Sometimes mood swing can increase suicidal thoughts among individual, idea of personal harm, risk taking behavior which can have detrimental effect on individual mental and physical well being.

Managing mood swings

These are the following strategies which can help an individual in managing mood swings effectively:

- **Tracking moods**: can aid in a better interpretation of emotional fluctuations and changes. Maintaining a written record of one's moods and journaling about them may assist some people in noticing trends in mood fluctuations and also potential triggers.
- **Exercise:** releases endorphins, which are stress-relieving substances that also enhance mood. Even light exercise can help to alleviate mood swings that occur frequently or unexpectedly.
- **Keeping a routine might be beneficial**. Doing tasks at the same time all day can help you manage your emotions.
- **Sleep** can help you feel better. Sleep deprivation can influence appetite and energy levels, as well as cause depression, anger, and an overall lack of happiness.
- **Nutrition** is regarded as an important factor in mood regulation. Getting sufficient nutrients and avoiding excessive sugar, liquor, and caffeine use may help to lessen the occurrence of mood swings.

Because mood swings can have a big impact on your health and well-being, specifically if the cause isn't addressed, seeking help from a mental health expert may be a good idea. Bipolar and depression, as well as other mood disorders, can be debilitating, and therapy sometimes can help deal with mood swings. Because mood swings are a symptom of an underlying disease rather than a diagnosable condition, the mental health expert will work with the individual in treatment to figure out what's causing them. In therapy, a person learns methods to manage mood swings that occur unexpectedly. Once this is done, it may be simpler to address the real issues using strategies like journaling, mindfulness, meditation, or breathing exercises.

A therapist often can assist a person in determining if mood swings arise as a result of such a mental health illness or as a sign of another type of worry. Whether mood swings arise as a consequence of mental or emotional suffering or are particular to a scenario, therapy may frequently aid in the process of recognising the reasons of highs and lows, and also situations that can lead one's mood to fluctuate. Individuals can also benefit from therapy to help them develop coping techniques for dealing with pressures as they emerge. In therapy, with the overall goal of learning to manage moods productively and maintain a good emotional balance, one can also learn to focus more on the present moment.

Mood swings and psychological disorders

Even though DSM-IV had a section on mood disorders, DSM-5, has just been updated to include separate categories on bipolar disorders and depressive disorders, which are commonly indicated by mood swings. While a persistently poor mood is frequently indicative of clinical depression, mood changes can also be an indicator. A manic episode, like those observed in bipolar disorder, can cause euphoric emotions, thoughts of invincible or grandiosity, as well as moods which lead to reckless behaviour or keep a person sleepless for days. When one's mood swings from high to low and back, it could be a sign of bipolar disorder.

One of the main goals of treatment is to treat or resolve mood issues without the use of medication wherever possible. However, some folks find that even a combination of medicine and counselling is the most effective way to keep severe mood swings from interfering with everyday living and function. Bipolar disorder, for example, is frequently treated with a combination of medication and treatment.

Impulsivity

Impulsive actions are a hallmark of BPD, as per the DSM-5, APA. In reality, it is the disorder's instability that best defines BPD. People with BPD frequently experience feelings of inadequacy, which manifest as unstable emotions, behaviours, and relationships. They may also be fast to react out at what they perceive to be insignificant issues, and they frequently fail to realize how illogical or overwhelming their feelings are.

Impulsive behaviours are innately inappropriate in psychological terms, whether that is in terms of scale or significant threat. A person with BPD is less likely to consider the consequences of their actions and is more likely to self-harm as a coping mechanism (such as binge eating or excessive drinking)

Impulsive behaviours, on the other hand, are not indicative of BPD by themselves. Only if a person's behaviour is pervasive, harmful, and interferes with their capacity to function normally may they be diagnosed with BPD (American Psychiatric Association).

Impulsivity is not to be confused with such a compulsion, which is characterised by abnormal behaviour that cannot be halted by a person who recognises it. The individual acts impulsively without realising that his or her behaviour is odd.

Diagnostic Criteria for BPD

BPD isn't the only condition that causes impulsive conduct. They're also linked to the following things:

➢ Physical reasons of impulsivity, such as a brain trauma or a neurodegenerative disease such as Alzheimer's or Huntington's disease;

➢ Bipolar mania, which is frequently accompanied with grandiosity as well as a flight of ideas. (When in an intense manic episode, an individual will frequently act rashly and without regard for the consequences.) Impulsivity linked to bipolar disease can manifest itself in a variety of ways, including shopping sprees and hypersexual activities (Zimmerman M and Morgan TA, 2013).

➢ Hyperactive-impulsive ADHD is a type of attention-deficit hyperactivity disorder (ADHD) characterised by a child's inability to sit still or regulate improper conduct. (It is this lack of control, combined with a continually shifting focus of interest, that causes impulsivity) (Miller DJ, et al., 2010).

➢ Substance use disorders, despite the fact that impulsivity is most often displayed while under the effect of drugs, when wanting drugs, or when actively pursuing drugs (Perry JL and Carroll ME., 2008).

> Antisocial personality disorder (ASPD), which is similar to BPD but differs in that it is characterised by a pervasive and persistent disrespect for morals, social standards, and other people's rights and feelings.

Twin studies have revealed that genetics likely play a larger influence in BPD than previously thought. A chromosome 9 genetic defect is thought to be linked to BPD symptoms, particularly the relative inheritability of impulsive aggression (Bornovalova, M.A., 2013). These mutations can affect the generation of dopamine and serotonin, the mood and cognition-related neurotransmitters, which are otherwise normal. According to Vanderbilt University research, impulsivity in the brain may also be connected to dopamine receptors in persons with BPD (Buckholtz J.W., et. al., 2016).

"Think things through" is a phrase that means "think things through."

BPD patients frequently experience depression-like sensations of emptiness and self-loathing, which could be explained by the same malfunctioning receptors. Without the ability to efficiently receive and transmit dopamine signals, a person's ability to retain self-control and emotional well-being is harmed (Buckholtz J.W., et. al., 2016).

This perfect storm of environmental, genetic, and physiological factors is likely to lead to the development of impulsivity in people with BPD and BPD.

Treatment of the Impulsivity

Although impulsive behaviours could be severe and pervasive, they can typically be addressed with treatment. Many BPD treatments include aspects that target impulsivity specifically.

Psychotherapy

DBT (dialectical behavioural therapy) focuses on establishing skills that reduce impulsive behaviour and increase your capacity to think and analyze before acting. By employing coping techniques to regulate powerful emotions, an individual with BPD is better ready to approach problems without conflict (May JM, 2016).

Mindfulness is a technique taught in DBT that makes it feel in the present moment, that can help you be more aware of your actions and contemplate the repercussions. Using this strategy can assist you in taking the time to think on your decisions, ability to make more sensible decisions about how to react to events in your environment. Mindfulness meditation is a popular strategy for promoting training (May JM, 2016).

Medication

Selected serotonin reuptake inhibitors (SSRIs), sometimes in combination with such a low antipsychotic dose, may also benefit. This is especially true if your behaviour is excessive and jeopardises your safety or the safety of people around you (May JM, 2016). Atypical antipsychotics, such as Abilify (aripiprazole), have been shown to lessen impulsivity and interpersonal issues.

Mood stabilisers: Lamictal (lamotrigine) and Topamax (topiramate) are two medications that can help with impulsivity, rage, and anxiety (Ripoll, L.H., 2013).

Coping

In addition to adhering to your therapeutic process and attending a therapist, there are things you may do to cope better with impulsivity. The very first step is usually to identify the inappropriate behaviour that you really want to change. Then, anytime you feel compelled to indulge in one of the other behaviours, use one of the following strategies:

- Analyze your behavior for misconduct and impulsivity. Try to control your emotions, thoughts, and outward actions.
- Try not to be too sensitive to any kind of personal problem.
- Engage yourself in social activity and try to make good contact with people of a particular social group.
- Try to speak frankly with your family members regarding day to day life problem which you are facing.
- Substitute your unhealthy behavior with a more healthy behavior.
- Try to be as optimistic as you can.

- ➢ Make a habit of doing physical exercise and psychological exercise i.e. meditation on a daily basis.
- ➢ Some of the effective techniques can also help you in coping like muscle relaxation exercises.
- ➢ Try to be more empathetic towards others.

Empathy

According to Hodges and Myers, empathy is generally defined as "understanding the experience of some other person by picturing oneself in that other person's circumstances." One knows the other person's experience as if he were going through it himself, but even without actually going through it.

Empathy is a moral building block which must reside within a doctor, and it is an absolute requirement. Being able to empathise with a patient's feelings allows a doctor to deliver more high quality care and put the patient more at ease throughout treatment. According to studies, the doctor's empathy has an impact on the patient's psychological characteristics and immunity.

According to Reiss, empathy serves a key personal and societal function by letting people to share their experiences, needs, and wishes while also serving as an emotional bridges that promotes pro-social behaviour (2017). However, research demonstrate that empathy decreases during medical school. Without focused treatments, uncompassionate treatment and care devoid of empathy leads in patients who really are dissatisfied. Then, when it comes to treatment suggestions, individuals are significantly less inclined to follow through, leading to a lower health outcomes and a loss of trust in medical professionals. Cognitive empathy must be used when there is a lack of emotional empathy owing to racial, cultural, religious, or physical disparities. Patients who vary from the majority group or the majority cultures of healthcare practitioners have really no place for discrimination or uneven care in healthcare environments, which are rife with conscious and unconscious biases.

There is still more work to be done to make healthcare more equal for healthcare practitioners and recipients of all cultures. Empathy for oneself and others results in the replenishment and renewal of a key human capacity. If we want to progress toward a more empathic society and a much more compassionate world, it is evident that we must develop individual, national, community, and global bonds in order to improve our natural empathy capacities.

Clinical empathy is a key component of high-quality care, and it has been associated to treatment adherence, higher patient satisfaction, and fewer malpractice complaints. According to Halpern (2012), empathy in medicine is difficult since doctors deal with some of the most emotionally painful events, such as illness, dying, and suffering in all forms, and such scenarios would normally make an empathic person nervous, possibly too anxious to be helpful. Burnout, detachment, and a low feelings of mastery may occur in physicians who are the most vulnerable to compassion fatigue and emotional distress, but the capacity to interact in self-other awareness one's emotions is critical to clinical practice's dynamic experience of empathy. These issues need to be investigated further because the medical profession tries to strike a good balance between job happiness and compassionate care.

Work related quality of life

The favorability or unfavourability of the workplace environment for those doing work in an company is referred to as work quality of life. During the era of scientific management, which was entirely focused on specialization and efficiency, a dramatic shift occurred. Human values have received little emphasis in traditional management (such like scientific leadership). Staff requirements and goals are shifting in the current environment. Employers are now redesigning jobs to improve QWL.

Quality of working life (QoWL) is a hypothetical concept which tries to explain an individual's satisfaction at workplace and his/her pleasurable experiences. The direct and indirect elements that affect an individual's QoWL, such like satisfaction at job and other features like workplace environment, relations with subordinates have an effect on their QoWL (Danna & Griffin, 1999). Enhancement in the subjective quality of work life have been linked to a number of benefits. Somerset County Council in the United Kingdom, for example, conducted a study to increase their employees' QoWL in order to reduce workplace stress and sickness absence. The ensuing reduction in worker sickness absence was predicted to yield a total net save of £1.57 million over two years.

A work design theory is a concept of job characteristics. It lays out *"a set of implementation principles for the economic gain of jobs within organizational context."* The original form of this theory includes five "core "characteristics of a job which can be named as-

1)   Skill Variety

2)   Role Clarity

3)   Task Significance

4)   Autonomy

5)   Feedback

These five core characteristics impact five work related outcomes-

1)   Motivation

2)   Satisfaction

3)   Performance

4)   Turnover

5)   Absenteeism

It also influences three psychological states-

1)   Experienced Responsibility

2)   Meaningfulness

3)   Knowledge of result

Working just under eight shifts a month but less than 80 hours a week were found to have a potential link with optimal work-life quality (QWL). Residents and organizations should be better managed in order to have the right number of working hours and to improve work-life balance, working conditions, general well-being, as well as job-career satisfaction. Workplace stress, from the other side, must always be minimized.

Work-life balance belongs to the good handling of many assignments at work, at homes, and in other areas of life. It's a problem that both employers and employees care about. Employees' views about being able using a flexibility in work hours programs to balance their employment and other duties such as family, interests, art, travel, studies, and so on, rather than only focused on work, are referred to as work life balance. This shows that a strong work-life balance leads to activities that increase employee satisfaction that make them valuable contributors to performance of the organization. A good work-life balancing is defined as a condition in which employees believe they can balance their job and non-work commitments.

Improving the efficiency of work-life balance service not only boosts productivity, but it also boosts employee loyalty and happiness. Employee attitudes toward their organisations, as well as their personal lives, are influenced by the work-life balance. Employee happiness, as well as organisational commitment and intention to stay with the organisation, are positively influenced by the notion that now the organisation cares for the well-being of its employees.

The work-life balance research includes information on the factors which enhances healthy work-life balance, the link between work-life alignment and satisfaction at job, the benefits of a healthy work-life balance, organizational strategies for balancing work and personal life, as well as employee awareness and preferences. positive job satisfaction,

Work motivation, enhanced morale and productivity of employees, adequate time for family responsibilities, improved health conditions, and so on are all good effects of proper Work Life Balance. Job stress, high attrition rate, work-life conflicts, burnouts, job switching, absenteeism, work drinking, health problems, and other indicators have all been linked to the detrimental effects of a work-life imbalance.

The term "work-family conflict" is used to describe a sort of inter-role conflict where at least some work and home duties are incompatible and have an impact to every field (Greenhaus & Beutell, 1985). Employee productivity, turnover, contentment, motivation, morale, and commitment to the organization could all be affected by this dispute.

Variables relating to persons, work-related variables, and family variables all influence an employee's work-life balance. Individual variables include sex, age, marital status, emotional wellbeing, and so on. Work-related variables include task diversity, task autonomy, work schedule flexibility, role conflict, amount of hours done, and so on. Support in spouses, workhours for spouses, job status of partners, number of kids, parenting responsibilities, domestic duties, and so on are all family-related variables.

Employees' reactions to work-life balance has major ramifications for businesses, employees, and organizations, according to previous research findings. Hobson, Delunas, and Kesic (2001), talked about the consequences of social and personal work life imbalance:

➢ Increased in intensity of stress related illness,
➢ Satisfaction of life at lower level,
➢ Physical aggression including violent behavior leading to divorce and family conflict,
➢ Drug addiction and alcoholic behavior,
➢ Problem in parenting and not able to provide sufficient timing to childrens,
➢ Juvenile criminality and violence are on the rise.

There are many unhealthy organizational consequences if an employee is not able to concentrate fully and is not willingly giving his personal best (Hobson, Delunas, and Kesic (2001):

➢ Absenteeism from workplace,
➢ Higher turnover intention,
➢ Lower productivity at workplace,
➢ Low level of satisfaction at job,
➢ Organization commitment and loyalty are lower,
➢ The cost of healthcare is increasing.

The advantages of having a work-life balance A good business plan must include positive work-life outcomes for people. Both the employee as well as the employer benefit when the correct balance is discovered and maintained.

Benefits for the employee:

- Many variables increase when an employee is capable of striking the correct balance.

- Some of these influences, as per Vlems (2005), include: Increased employee contentment: Employees will be happier if they could balance their job and personal obligations.

- Improved management relationships: Employees' perceptions of getting support from management for work-life balance build a positive association between workforce and management, which enhances internal communication.

- Workers self esteem can be boosted, it can also increase awareness and attentiveness,

- Building of a self-trust,

- Employee loyalty as well as dedication: These factors contribute to a better work-life balance.

- Employees are more inclined to stay with a company if there are options to establish a work-life balance.

- Motivation increases, tasks are superior managed, and the level of stress between employees decreases.

Benefits for the employer

According to Vlems (2005), the following factors enhance for the employer:

- **Maximized accessible labour**: The workers will be extremely motivated, allowing the company to gain from maximised available labour. During working hours, each employee will do his or her absolute best.

- **Employees feel valued because of the balance**: Work-life balance programmes are implemented to convey the appearance that the corporation cares about its employees. As just a result, individuals will value themselves more and work more. The working atmosphere will be less distressing, resulting in fewer illnesses and lower health-care costs.

- **Employer of choice:** When it comes to employment, having work-life balance policies in place makes a company more appealing to a wider spectrum of individuals. Increased employee loyalty and reduced absenteeism: Employees will become more faithful more motivated, absenteeism will decrease, and efficiency will rise with time.

CHAPTER – 2

REVIEW OF LITERATURE

It is vital for the researcher to investigate and discuss similar research undertaken by other researchers afterwards discussing and establishing the theoretical backdrop of the study. This research endeavor builds on all previous relevant thinking and study, forms part of the field's acquired expertise, and contributes to overall body of knowledge. The review of related literature in this chapter is addressed.

Reviews related to Quality of sleep

The study's goal, according to Keller (2001), is to determine whether sleep disorders in chronically sick patients are connected with decreased functional health and the well, decreased work functioning, and increased the use health services. A cross sectional study was conducted based on survey method related to patients in which focus was on health and wellbeing. It was observed form the study that significant changes were seen between patients having sleep disorder and those who are free from these kinds of symptoms.

When compared to physical health indicators, measures of mental wellbeing and the mental health overview were most linked with sleep problem severity in the entire sample and chronic disease subsets, according to the relative effect analysis. Furthermore, there has been a consistent link discovered between the complexity of sleep difficulties and decreased work productivity and increased health-care utilisation.. Sleep issues are linked to poor mental health, decreased productivity and quality of work, and higher usage of health services, according to the findings. As a result, sleep issues may have a role in the interpreting of health outcomes in chronic disease patients.

Burgard and Ailshire (2009) research uses the Changing Lives study of longitudinal and nationally representative Americans to examine whether and how common working conditions and experiences can "follow workers home" and affect their sleep quality. It also explores how competing stressful experiences at home can affect the quality of sleep, and whether these are more important than experiences at work. Results show that being bothered or upset at work frequently is associated with poorer quality of sleep, and stressful experiences at home.

Luz & Tubaro (2011) Nursing technicians as well as assistants who served 12-hour night shifts at the a charity hospital were studied to see if there was a link between job happiness and sleep quality. This study included 81 professionals, with an average lifespan of 31.9 years. Sleep disturbance was associated with female gender.

The study's goal, according to Momeni (2016), is to assess the association between work quality and sleeping in nurses working in ICUs in Iran's Mazandaran province. At 2015, 180 nurses working in teaching hospital ICUs affiliated with the University of Medical Sciences of Mazandaran, Iran, participated in this cross-sectional, descriptive-correlational study. In this study, ICU nurses were unsatisfied with the majority of characteristics related to work life quality. Furthermore, 49 respondents had a bad QOWL, while 119 and 12 cases, respectively, had a moderate and excellent quality of work life. It was also revealed that 69 and 111 nurses, respectively, had good and poor sleep quality. The quality of work life as well as the quality of sleep were found to have a substantial, inverse, linear relationship. According to the findings of this study, the majority of ICU nurses' work life as well as sleep quality were average and unfavourable, respectively. In moreover, the quality of one's sleep was linked to the quality of one's professional life.

The goal of Fernandes-Junior (2016) is to assess night shift employees' sleep duration, exhaustion, and quality of life, and even the relationship between the variables and the presence and absence of children in various age groups. Conclusion was that during working days, workers without children had greater sleep time. These employees were also less likely than workers with children to feel tired during night work, regardless of the age of these children.

De Carvalho (2018) study's objective is to evaluate sleep quality, QoL and mood disorders in central hospital healthcare providers. Sleep disorders among healthcare providers that impair circadian rhythm, neurobehavioral functions and quality of life are common (QoL). The study enrolled 108 professionals of which

66.7% were poor sleepers. Most subjects worked rotating night shifts in both groups and had poor hygiene for sleep, but denied excessive daytime sleepiness (EDS). Poor sleepers had longer mean latency for sleep, more symptoms of insomnia, shorter mean duration of sleep, higher daytime dysfunction, higher mean anxiety and depression scores and worse overall QoL perception. Poor sleep quality was associated with mood disorders and poorer perceived QoL in our study. Although without EDS, most subjects had poor sleep hygiene in both groups, which may gradually worsen the quality of sleep even in good sleepers. Providing them with conditions to enhance their sleep and well-being is crucial.

Kim is a student at the University of (2018) The goal of the study was to determine the sleep habits of daylight employees that do not work at night. The study looked into the factors that affect sleep length and quality. Or more a thousand day workers were studied in this study belonging to manufacturing profession. A self-administered questionnaire was taken to study demographic factors including working time, quality of job, motor symptoms etc. to evaluate sleep behavior. Regular health checks were conducted as part of the worker's clinical checkup. Sleep length was linked to the type of employment and obesity.

Lim (2018) conducted a study in order to examine the health related quality of work life (HRQoL) of those workers who are doing night shifts on a daily basis. Age range of employees varied from 40 to 65 years and this sample was compared with non-workers in a cross-sectional survey of manufacturing facilities in Malaysia. Sleep deprivation and poor HRQoL were linked to night-shift work, according to the findings. When both the groups were compared, the results were found to be shocking as it showed a poor quality of health among workers doing nigh shifts and vice versa. There was also a disturbance of sleep cycle among night shift employees. It can be concluded from these kind of studies that organization should take some initiative to improve the quality of work life among workers.

Deng, Liu, and Fang (2020) Chronic sleep deprivation can exacerbate a variety of physiological and mental health disorders, making it difficult to operate well at work. In a general hospital, job stress might be a factor that significantly correlates with decreased sleep quality for nurses from various departments. In China, there are few epidemiological studies of sleep difficulties among nurses, and no studies of the link between sleep issues and professional stress. This study looked into the relationship between nurses' job stress and sleep quality in a regional hospital in China.

This cross-sectional study included 180 nurses who had worked for even more than a year in 12 community hospitals. Sleep disruptions were associated with the type of nursing contracts and total occupational stress levels. Sleep quality was found to be adversely correlated with work stress levels, implying that the higher job stress level, the poorer the sleep quality. The form of nursing contracts and self-reported occupational stress were found to be key factors that affect sleep quality in the logistic regression study. Nurses' sleep disturbances were highly linked to job difficulty, doctor-patient connections, psychosomatic condition, surroundings or events, promotion as well as competition, or total pressure scores.

Reviews related to Mood swings

Pugliesi (1999) Early research suggested that emotional labour performance had deleterious effects on employees, but recent empirical research has been misleading. Emotional labour performance appears to have various consequences for workers, both negative and positive. The diverse modes of emotion regulation may account for the heterogeneity inside the effects of emotional labour. Other job factors may also influence the impacts of emotional labour, according to studies. Employees are universally negatively affected by both types of emotional work, gross of work complexity, management, and demands, according to the findings. Emotional labour raises job stress perceptions, decreases job satisfaction, and raises distress. The effects of self-focused emotion management are the most persistent and detrimental. There is very little evidence that work conditions but also emotional labour have an impact on interaction.

The goal of Woo & Postolache's (2008) paper was to examine the evidence for calculating the effect of occupational characteristics on mood and suicidal disorders, as well as the efficacy of therapies. This evaluation is based on the observation of previous studies conducted between 1966 and 2007 using Medline as well as Psych INFO. To establish a link between occupational characteristics and mood disorders, we focused on clinically significant illnesses rather than depressive symptoms. It has been revealed from epidemiological studies that occupational characteristics and mood disorder are positively related.

Workers' access to therapy is still limited due to a lack of awareness and social stigma. Mental health specialists must collaborate with companies to develop a creative system that makes high-quality services accessible to employees.

Cheung and Tang (2009) used the resource conservation model to investigate the links between emotional labour, work family interference, and work quality of life. 442 Chinese service employees in Hong Kong provided self-reported data for a cross-sectional study. Even though the principles of organisational display or demographic data of employees were controlled, the results of correlation with hierarchical regression analysis revealed that surface behaviour has a substantial correlation with work-to-family interference. Furthermore, the quality of work life mediated the association across surface action but also work-to-family interference. This study gave vital information about how to apply various emotional labour methods in relation to working family interference. Based on our findings, significant acting inside the workplace should really be encouraged because it was linked to a higher QOW'L but did not exacerbate work-family conflict. While previous research has looked at emotional labour as a prelude to work family interference, ours was one of the first to look at family-to-work interference as an emotional labour backdrop. Furthermore, research was proven that the role of work-life quality is an essential mediator of emotional work-family conflict.

Carvalho (2017) discusses the issues of Quality of Working Life (QWL) as well as Occupational Stress, with the goal of proposing an exploratory study to investigate how these topics have been addressed in a developing country like Brazil.

A persistent search towards goals or outcomes began, putting more pressure on the workplace and resulting in a huge number of workplace accidents, in addition to increased employee stress. While there is evidence of a link between workplace conditions and illnesses, it remains difficult to fully comprehend and analyse this issue. The purpose of this study was to see if there is a link between quality of working life with occupational stress, and if so, how we may reduce stress in the workplace by implementing QWL.

Reviews related to Impulsivity

Grant & Chamberlain (2019) Impulsive and compulsive behaviors are common in young adulthood, which would be a vital period for cognitive development and defining life objectives. The goal of this study was to find crucial links between impulsivity and compulsivity and quality of life among young adults using a variety of clinical, questionnaire, as well as cognitive measures. Older age, higher alcohol consumption, and the presence of impulse control disorders, post-traumatic stress disorder, mood/anxiety disorders and drug use disorder were all associated with lower quality of life variables.

Al-Masri (2020) wanted to see if there was a link between impulsive purchase behaviour and emotional balance among students from Petra University Accounting Department and Al-Imam Mohammad Ibn Saud Islamic University, based on nationality, gender, and economic status. The study discovered a negative relationship between impulsive purchasing and emotional equilibrium.

Reviews related to Empathy

Hirsch (2007) instructors emphasized the importance of empathy throughout medical school, usually defined as the understanding of and identification with the emotional state of another person. Commonly confused with each other, sympathy and empathy are not the same. Sympathy is a declaration of emotional concern, while empathy reflects emotional comprehension.

Empathy applications are widespread, and are particularly relevant in fields such as medicine, where effective patient-physician interactions depend on the successful treatment of patients. From the perspective of a medical student, this article explored the concept of empathy and examines its usefulness in medicine.

Decety & Gleichgerrcht (2013) A large-scale study including 7,584 board - certified plastic practitioners was done to understand better clinical empathy and also what factors can sabotage its experience and consequence in care-giving settings. Empathic concern, perspective taking, and altruism were all substantially linked to compassion satisfaction. Physicians who struggle with negative arousal regulation and who appear to be more susceptible to emotional weariness, detachment, and a weak sense of accomplishment to express and identify feelings.

Paro (2014) aimed to evaluate the empathy of medical students and their associations with gender, medical school stage, quality of life and burnout. A total of 1,650 students were selected at random, out of which all questionnaires were completed only by 1,350 (81.8%). Female students showed greater empathic dispositional concern as well as experienced more personal distress than their male counterparts. There were slight discrepancies in the empathetic settings of students at various phases of their medical education. Depersonalization was linked to a decrease in empathetic concern and viewpoint taking. Higher perspective taking and lower personal distress scores were associated with personal achievement. There were greater empathic concern and personal distress arrangements for female students.

Chan is a Chinese character (2015) Burnout and compassion fatigue have recently been identified as occupational hazards in the medical field. Burnout, dedication to work, compassion fatigue, and fulfillment among doctors were all investigated in our study. Self-efficacy, kind of robust personality, sense of thankfulness, and calling for work were all investigated in relation to these four quantifiable intrinsic human variables. The study discovered a weak but significant negative link between burnout with participation, as well as a bad negative correlation between compassion fatigue and satisfaction. Burnout, job engagement, compassion fatigue, and satisfaction were significantly correlated with only intrinsic human factors. Our preliminary results indicate that certain intrinsic variables increase the commitment to work and the satisfaction of compassion among doctors.

Agarwal, Agarwal, Agarwal, A (2017) In simple terms, empathy entails experiencing someone person's emotions and determining what they are thinking or feeling. The goal of this study was to see if there was a difference in empathy, compassion, but also quality of life between nursing and medical students. Another goal of the research was to look into the link among empathy, compassion, but also quality of life between nursing and medical students. The findings revealed that there was a difference in empathy, compassion, quality of life, and its components of physical health and surroundings between nursing and medical students. Empathy was positively connected with quality of life in nursing students, but was adversely correlated to quality of life in medical students. These findings are pertinent to patients' hospital experiences as well as the clinician-patient interaction.

Cánovas (2018) studied to study the impact on pain relief and HR-QoL of the empathy of doctors perceived by patients with chronic pain. A prospective non-interventional study was conducted on 2898 patients who were referred to pain clinics with moderate to severe chronic pain. At the baseline and after one and three months, the same physician visited each patient. Regression analyses were used to determine the unique contribution of changes in viewed empathy to improvements in HR-QoL. Physician empathy and patient dispositional optimism both have a role in deciding positive outcomes in chronic pain patients. Physician empathy may thus be an appropriate, although largely untapped, target for intervention.

Keshavarz (Keshavarz) is a Persian (2019) The professional QOL is an important component that everyone considers in their employment. The purpose of this study was to assess health care providers' professional quality of life and related characteristics (doctors, nurses, and midwives). In 2018, a convenience sample of 464 doctors, nurses, and midwives working in Qazvin University of Medical Sciences teaching hospitals were studied in a cross-sectional study. Medium and high job satisfaction, monthly salary, and work shift agreements were all major variables in the regression model for all categories of professional quality of life. As a result, it has the potential to improve health-care providers' professional quality of life, hence the quality of patient treatment.

Moudatsou's current work (2020) is an integrative but also analytical literature study on the idea and meaning of empathy among health and social care professionals. Health care providers that have a high level of empathy have been demonstrated to be more effective in their function in inducing therapeutic change. The enormous number of patients whom professionals must manage, the lack of enough time, and the current academic culture's emphasis on therapy all have a negative impact on the development of empathy.

The development of empathic abilities should be a primary goal of not only undergraduate health and social care education, but also lifetime and continual professional education.

Reviews related to Quality of Work Life

Hackman and Oldham (1976) brought attention to what they called "psychological growth requirements" as being relevant to the quality of work life. Several such demands were found, including skill variation, task identity, task relevance, autonomy, and feedback. These demands, it was stated, must be met if the employees are to have a high quality of work life.

A study was conducted on secondary school teachers and principals to see their quality of work life. It was found that Principals were shown to have a good influence on teacher respect, teacher engagement in choices affecting their job, professional collaboration as well as interaction, application of knowledge, and thus the learning environment (Rossmiller, 1992).

Eaton (1992) investigated the impact of a QOWL programme and grievance mechanisms on union membership. This was determined based on the analysis data data from a 1987 poll of four separate bargaining units in same local union. The researchers discovered that the perceived efficacy of the grievance system influenced sentiments toward the union far more than participation in a quality of work life programme. It led the authors to speculate that improving the effectiveness of the grievance procedure could be one way for unions to strengthen their ties with their members.

Lam (1995) studied the links between work life quality, career commitment, job satisfaction, and withdrawal cognition in 350 Singapore teacher trainees. The findings revealed that teachers' evaluations of their social status were substantially linked to their dedication and happiness in the classroom. The quality of work life and productivity were studied by Elmuti and Yunus Kathawala (1997). The influence of involvement in a self-managed group programme on personnel quality of work life attitudes, productivity, and quality was researched among employees in a manufacturing company in the midwestern United States.

The attitudinal findings demonstrate that self-managed teams improved the participant's work life quality. The self-managed group programme had a significant and beneficial influence on staff productivity, efficiency, and quality, as evidenced by the performance outcomes.

Mentz (2001) conducted research to determine the working conditions of educators residing in Africa. A total sample of 60 teachers belonging to 15 rural schools was taken for the present study. It was found from the research that teachers ar equite satisfied with their working conditions and they enjoy being sharing knowledge in rural areas. They liked the capacity of the classroom, the physical facilities, and the student-teacher connections.

Susan (2006) Harrington and Julie Santiago investigated the QOWL and professional isolation of telecommuters in the context of organisational culture. The relationship between job quality, professional isolation, and also the cultural values of an organization's telecommuters and non-telecommuters was investigated in this study. Telecommuting is more common in a far less hierarchical culture, according to the studies. In the rational culture, however, there was no discernible difference between telecommuters and nontelecommuters. Telecommuters had much higher quality of life or professional isolation than non-telecommuters, corroborating virtual worker literature as well as theory.

Lee, Dong-Jin (2007) Sirgy et al. created a need-based assessment of Quality of Work Life (QWL) that was studied and verified. They developed the QWL construct using two sets of major demands: lower- and higher-order needs, in terms of employee. Health/safety requirements but also family/economic demands are examples of lower-order requirements. Social needs, esteem needs, self-actualization needs, knowledge needs, and aesthetic needs are examples of higher-order requirements. As expected, QWL had a beneficial impact on organizational commitment and job satisfaction among marketing managers.

Dolan is a well-known figure in the (2007) In Catalonia, the factors of low job quality and bad health across primary health care workers were explored. The research was based on large-scale survey data from Catalonia's public health care system in 1995, 2002, and 2003, respectively. The research, on the other hand, used a cross-sectional methodology. The findings of the 2002 cross-sectional study back up stress researchers' claims that both job demands and a lack of supervisory assistance predict low QWL and negative health effects. Perceived motivation, resources, and capabilities are also determinants, albeit to a lesser amount. Because the study included all types of employees in the health-care industry, it had a high level of external validity. The findings enable tangible actions to be done to minimise stress, alleviate negative health effects, and improve the quality of people's working life in this industry.

Erickson (2008) investigated the working conditions of instructors of American Indian kids. The purpose of this study was to re-validate the QTWLS ("Quality of Teacher Work Life Survey") with a population of 404 instructors in Montana schools with a high percentage of American Indian students, as well as to describe the stress and happiness of those teachers at work. Factor analysis revealed nine satisfaction and eight stress components for this demographic in Pelsma, Richard, and Harrington's (1989) study with mostly Caucasian teachers and students, compared to eleven satisfaction and ten stress elements for the general population. Results of the QTWLS outcomes lead to interventions that contribute to an improved working life for American Indian student teachers and increased learning among students.

Soren Ventegodt (2008) A scientific study on the QWL was carried out, through a generic measurement of the global quality of working life with the questionnaire self-assessment of the quality of working life. Stress, job satisfaction, working environment, health, personal functioning, and immediate subjective well-being at work are all examples of good working life quality.

Ayodeji (2009) studied Job Design and improved Nigerian Secondary School teachers' quality of work life. This research focused on how the best job design could lead to Nigerian teachers improving the quality of work life. One of the conclusions drawn in the study was that an efficient job design could lead to better performance and satisfaction of employees, but there was no universally good job design. The relative effectiveness of the four approaches to job design was affected by individual differences, organisational climate, style, interpersonal relationships and the state of technology.

At an Industrial Vocational School in Taiwan, Chao and Yang (2010) investigated the association between principal leadership behaviour and teachers' work quality. An industrial vocational school in Taiwan was used as a case study. Second, all instructors at the industrial vocational school were polled about the principal's leadership style as well as the quality of their work environment.The findings showed the differences in the views of teachers with different backgrounds on the principal's leadership behaviour and the quality of work life, as well as the relationship between two variables.

Louis (2011) looked into how teachers' work-life quality affects their commitment to their jobs and perception of effectiveness. A model was given that connects organisational features of the workplace to essential instructors' behaviours, attitudes, and psychological factors that influence their teaching. The relationship in between QOWL different factors and the commitment and feeling of effectiveness of educators' measures was then investigated in eight schools, as well as the relationship in between quality of work life factors and the commitment and feeling of effectiveness of educators' measures. Finally, the impact of the structure of the school on the quality of working life was examined. The data indicated that work life quality measures are strongly associated with commitment as well as a sense of effectiveness.

Pisheh (2012) conducted a study with the goal of determining the association in between quality of work life and job stress among Iranian government employees.The cross sectional design was used for this descriptive design. In order to draw 200 employees from 24 public organisations in the township of Sirjan in Kerman province, a proportional cluster sampling method was used. Using two validated instruments, variables in the study were evaluated. To analyse the data, descriptive and inferential statistics were employed. The results of the investigation found that the quality of work life and work stress of public employees in Iran is correlated.

Hamidi and Mohamadi are two of the most well-known figures in the Islamic world (2012) The quality of work life rate between academic and technical high school teachers in the Iranian province of Kordestan was compared in a causal-comparative research study. Teachers in technical schools faced different integrations as well as differences from teachers at other theoretical schools in terms of organisation, work life and social dependency, and general living space, resulting in different growth chances. The study sample consisted of 410 high school teachers chosen through cluster sampling. They used the QWL questionnaire. It was observed that the Cronbach's Alpha reliability of the instrument was 0.98. Using descriptive and inferential statistics, the data was analysed.

The findings revealed that (a) Kordestan's technical and theoretical high school instructors had an average quality of working life, and (b) there was no significant association between the type of high school (technical or theoretical) and the quality of working life. The QWL of these two types of high school did not differ much, and the quality of working life in all theoretical and technical high schools of Kordestan was the same.

Indian Studies related to Quality of Work Life

Ganguli and Joseph (1976) of Air India investigated the quality of working life among young workers, with a focus on issues of life and job happiness. Different physical and psychological working conditions, pride in organisation, job earned community respect, and reasonable working hours were found to be positively correlated with job satisfaction rather than friendship with colleagues, variety of abilities, good workplace, physical strain, and risks of injury. Young workers' expectations and aspirations have also been found to influence their quality of working life.

Rao (1985) conducted research to see if there was a difference in the quality of work life among male and female employees who did similar jobs. Male employees had a considerably higher composites quality overall working life score than female employees, according to the findings. The ability to develop new abilities, workplace challenges, and discretionary work features were all much higher among men's employees. He discovered that women's working lives were judged to be of higher quality when they were older and had more money.

Suri (1991) conducted a survey to investigate the quality of work-life practises in India. Manufacturing and service industries were the focus of the study. The findings of the study revealed a number of trends that had consequences for Quality of Work Life practises and outcomes. Job and workplace transformation programmes were disliked by both government and non - governmental enterprises. Rather than isolated experiments limited to certain areas or departments, organisations favoured system-wide methods.

More than 200 instructors were given two structured questionnaires designed specifically for the study to assess their current as well as expected Quality of Work Life. The present and predicted Quality of Work Life of Sardar Patel University instructors were found to be significantly different. But in the case of Maharaja Sayajirao University, lecturers were expecting improvement in Quality of Work Life.

Mohanraj (2010) aimed to assess the state of QWL in NTC mills in Tamil Nādu, as well as how QWL contributes to a healthy and robust work culture. QWL was defined in this study as enough and fair compensation in the workplace, safe and hygienic workplace circumstances, and social integration which allows the individual to grow and use all of his or her potential. The goal of the study was to determine the role of QWL among NTC mill employees in sustaining a positive work environment. To collect primary data, a well-structured, unmasked questionnaire was used. This study revealed some good elements of QWL, with the major finding being that employees of different statuses had different preferences for QWL factors.

The findings of the study showed that flexi-working circumstances and alternate work schedules were highly anticipated. Employees had a particular perspective on QWL facets, and they were quite unsatisfied with the availability of specific QWL facets, including such welfare measures, recognition, and work conditions. To establish a robust work culture, many aspects of QWL were provided to employees in various positions, as well as strengthening interpersonal connections, participatory management, and physical working conditions.

A study on the quality of working life just like perceived by college instructors was undertaken by Burethina, Subburethina, and Bharathi (2011). This study looked at the quality of college professors' working life from a variety of perspectives. This research helped college teachers to understand and improve the level of perception of QWL by educational administrators. 12 colleges located in the city of Tiruchirappalli and 1279 college teachers worked from May 2008 to February 2009 were part of the study universe. From the universe, a sample of 239 respondents was selected. The link between the quality of one's work life . it includes of one's life in the classroom was discovered to be considerable. The QWL of university professors was discovered to be poor.

Kadhiravan & Parameswari (2011) Teachers from both public and private schools were researched to see if there was a link between both the quality of their work lives and their ability to self-regulate their behaviour. For this study, 60 school teachers (30 from the government and 30 from the private sector) were polled about their work life quality and self-control. The findings revealed that both government and private school instructors have a high level of job satisfaction and self-control. Certain work-life quality characteristics and self-regulated behaviour variables were found to be linked.

Indumathy, Induma, and Kamalraj (2012) investigated the quality of work life among workers in Tirupur District, a textile hub, with a focus on the textile industry. The study design that was adopted was descriptive. A total of 60 workers were picked using easy sampling. A systematic interview schedule was employed for the initial data gathering. Secondary data was acquired through previous research, as well as published journals, periodicals, websites, and online publications. The survey found that attitude, career prospects, difficulties, atmosphere, possibilities, people, nature of work, stress level, growth and development, and risk involved in work, as well as rewards, were the most important elements influencing and deciding the quality of work life.

Sinha (2012) conducted research into the factors that influence the quality of work-life experiences in organisations. The study looked at 100 employees in middle management positions from various companies. The three emerging variables were relationship-sustenance orientation, prospective and professional orientation, and self-deterministic as well as systemic orientation. The findings revealed that these variables play an important role in meeting employee needs, as well as how various facets were valued but also shown at the management level to create a unique quality of working life inside their socio-technical systems in order to generate positive job-related responses.

Gayathiri and Ramakrishnan (2013) looked into the quality of work life or how it relates to job satisfaction and job performance. An attempt is made in this study to evaluate the quality of life literature in addition to identifying concept and measurement factors, as well as their relationship to satisfaction and performance.

The impact of the quality of work life on employee retention in private sector banks has been studied. This study further explored that QWL not only contributed to the ability of a company to recruit quality people, but also improved the competitiveness of a company. The results indicated that QWL will positively nurture a more flexible, loyal and motivated workforce, as per common beliefs, which are essential in determining the competitiveness of the company.

CHAPTER – 3

RESEARCH METHODOLOGY

The chapter describes the method of study to fulfill the objectives and to test the hypotheses. The study aimed to explain the impact of quality of sleep, mood swings, impulsivity, and empathy in relation to work related quality of life among doctors. For any type of research, research design is important as it outlines how the research will be conducted, how it will guide and direct data collection, analysis of data and data reporting. For the present research correlational design was used.

Objectives:

- To investigate the association between quality of sleep, mood swings, impulsivity, empathy and work-related quality of life among doctors.
- To investigate the role of work-related quality of life on quality of sleep, mood swings, impulsivity and empathy among doctors.

Hypotheses:

- There would be positive relationship between quality of sleep and work related quality of life.
- There would be negative relationship between mood swings and work related quality of life.
- There would be a negative relationship between impulsivity and work related quality of life.
- There would be a positive relationship between empathy and work related quality of life.
- Quality of sleep would act as a significant contributor in Work related quality of life.
- Mood swings would act as a significant contributor in Work related quality of life.
- Impulsivity would act as a significant contributor in Work related quality of life.
- Empathy would act as a significant contributor in Work related quality of life.

Sample

The total sample for the present study was 300 resident doctors. The age of doctors were between 30-35 years, work experience of at least 5 years. The sample was selected from North India region, specifically Haryana, Punjab and NCR region.

Tools Used

The following standardized instruments were used for present investigation:

1)   Sleep Quality Scale
2)   Positive and Negative Affect schedule (PANAS)
3)   Barratt Impulsiveness Scale
4)   Empathy Quotient
5)   The Work related Quality of Life scale

Brief description of the tools:

Sleep Quality Scale (SQS):

This scale helps in examining six particular dimensions of SQS. It was developed in 2006. The scale is a basic self-report, pencil-and-paper assessment that takes between 5 and 10 minutes to administer. The sleep quality is measured on a four point Likert scale ranging from (0 = "few," 1="some-times," 2 = "often," and 3 = "nearly always"). Scoring of some of the items are in reversed format i.e. item 2 and 5. Raw score range falls in between 0 to 84. High score on sleep quality indicates serious sleep issues faced by an individual while low score indicates good quality sleep. The six subdimensions are following- daytime symptoms, restoration after sleep, issues starting and sustaining sleep, trouble awakening, and sleep satisfaction.

Positive and Negative Affect Schedule (PANAS):

The PANAS scale is developed by Watson in 1988 which includes a total of twenty items. This method is trustworthy and a valid procedure in which two type of mood states are evaluated throughout various time intervals ('today,' 'over the last few days,' 'during the previous year,' 'on average,' etc.) as positive and negative mood. The good feeling is measured on one scale, while the negative emotion is measured on the other.

Each segment has 10 words that may be assessed on a scale of 1 to 5 to indicate how much the responder agrees that the phrase pertains to him. With measures including overall distress and dysfunction, depression, and state anxiety, the PANAS has excellent reported validity.

Barratt Impulsiveness Scale:

It was created by Ernest Barratt and consists of 30 items that are scored to yield six first order factors and three second order factors (attention, motor, self control, cognitive complexity, perseverance, and cognitive instability impulsive (attentional, motor, and non-planning impulsiveness). A total score, three second-order factors and six first-order factors are calculated from the BIS. On a 4-point scale, items are graded rarely (1), occasionally (2), often (3), and always (4) (4).

Empathy Quotient (EQ):

It is a 60-item questionnaire meant to assess adult empathy. Simon Baron-Cohen of the University of Cambridge's ARC (Autism Research Centre) created the exam. The EQ empathy assessments are used by mental health specialists to determine the extent of social impairment; however, this questionnaire can also be used with normal population or general community. The EQ comprises of 60 items, 40 of which are empathy-related and 20 of which are not. A short version of this questionnaire is also available having only 40 items but is found to be less accurate in some of the conditions.

Each item is a first-person remark that must be rated as "strongly agree," "somewhat agree," or "slightly disagree", "strongly disagree" by the administrator. Responses has to be given in regard to each of the question given in a questionnaire, score range of a questionnaire can vary from 0 to 80. High score indicates least empathetic behavior and vice versa.

The Work-Related Quality of Life (WRQoL) scale:

This scale is developed by Kaston and Laar in 2012 in which there are total 23 items used to analyze employees subjective quality of life as evaluated by six psychosocial sub-factors. GWB (Overall Well-Being) measures psychological well-being as well as general physical health. HWI (Home-Work Interface) - Workplace Control WRQoL (CAW) - this subscale measures how engaged you feel in workplace choices that impact you. Working Circumstances (WCS) - This subscale determines how happy you are with your current working conditions. Stress at Job (SAW) - This subscale measures how acceptable work pressures and expectations are compared to how stressful they are.

Procedure

The samples were collected over the internet. After the instruments for the current study were finalised, the respondents were called for data collection, and a rapport was built by making them feel at ease. The respondents were then provided the surveys along with explicit instructions on how to complete them. The respondents were given enough time to read and complete the surveys. The data was analysed using Pearson product moment correlation after the questionnaires were collected.

Scoring and Statistical Analysis:

The acquired data was recorded for statistical analysis in order to meet the study's goals. All of the tests were scored according to the directions in the scoring handbook. To obtain the data for statistical analysis, correlational and regression analysis were used.

CHAPTER – 4

RESULTS

The results have been presented under the following headings:

A- Section I: Descriptive Statistics on tested variables (Mean & Standard Deviations)

B- Section II: Inter correlation among tested variables (Pearson Product Moment Coefficient of Correlation)

C- Section III: Regression Analysis (Stepwise Multiple Regression Analysis)

SECTION-I

(DESCRIPTIVE STATISTICS)

This section explains descriptive statistics i.e. mean and SD for the composite score and subscales of each variable. "Descriptive statistics are used to describe the basic features of the data in a study. They provide simple summaries about the sample and measures"........

For this purpose, descriptive statistics (mean & standard deviations) for all the variables and their subscales was calculated and represented graphically.

Table 4.1: Descriptive Statistics (mean & SD's) for doctors i.e. (N=300)

	Mean	Standard Deviation	N
Quality of sleep	39.21	12.79	300
Positive emotions	33.34	4.25	300
Negative emotions	16.24	3.76	300
Impulsivity	66.10	7.14	300
Empathy	50.50	10.63	300
General well being	22.59	3.75	300
Homework interface	10.96	1.83	300
Job and satisfaction	22.94	4.37	300
Control at work	10.30	1.74	300
Working conditions	10.44	1.37	300
Stress at work	6.34	1.21	300
Work related Quality of Life	77.20	6.78	300

From Table 1: it can be observed that quality of sleep mean score was 39.21(SD= 12.79). For the positive emotions the mean score was 33.34 (SD=4.25). On negative verbal aggression subscale mean score was found to be 16.24 (SD=3.76). Impulsivity had a mean score of 66.10 (SD= 7.14). Empathy had a mean score of 50.50 (SD=10.63).

From the table 1: it can also be observed that General well-being, Homework interface, Job and satisfaction, Control at work, Working conditions, Stress at work sub dimensions of work related quality of life For the General well-being the mean score was 22.59 (SD=3.75). On homework interface subscale mean score was found to be 10.96 (SD= 1.83). Job and satisfaction had a mean score of 22.94 (SD= 4.37). Control at work had a mean score of 10.30 (SD=1.74). working conditions had a mean score of 10.44 (SD= 1.37). Stress at work had a mean score of 6.34 (SD= 1.21 The overall scale i.e. Work related quality of life had a mean score of 77.20 (SD= 6.78).

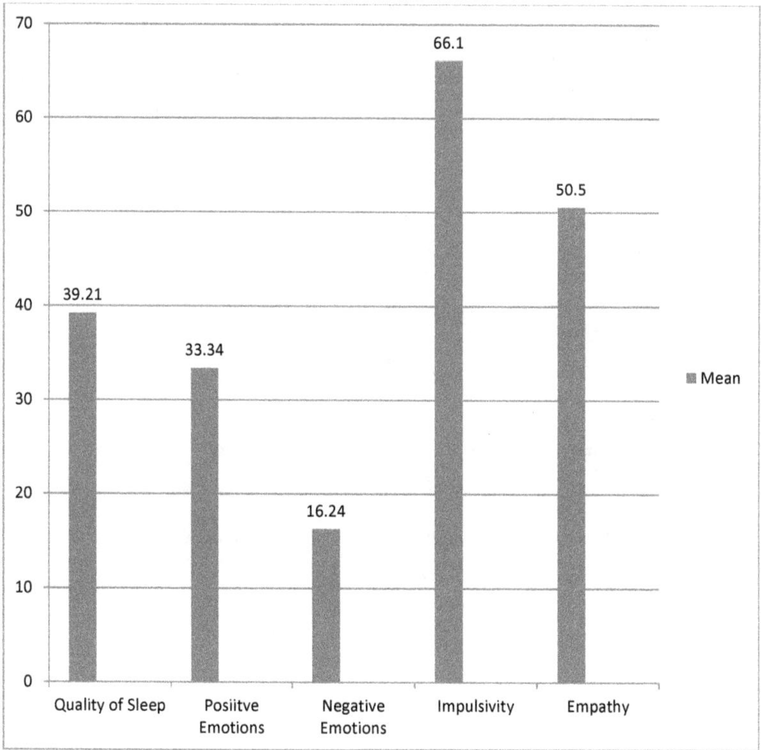

Figure 4.1: *Mean scores for quality of sleep, positive emotions, negative emotions, impulsivity and empathy are shown (N=300).*

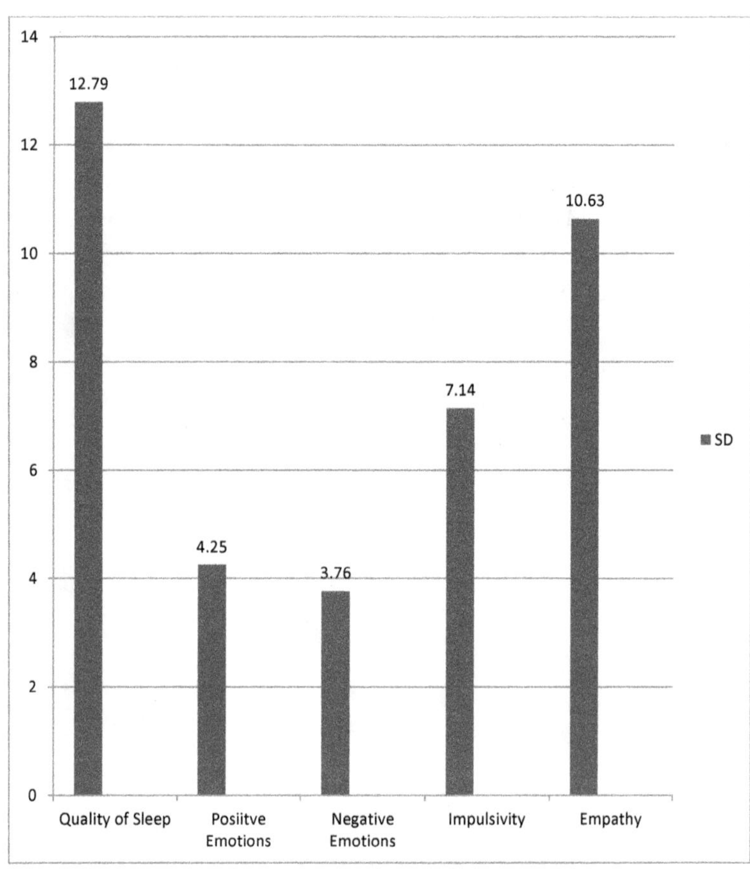

Figure 4.2: SD's scores for quality of sleep, positive emotions, negative emotions, impulsivity and empathy are shown (N=300).

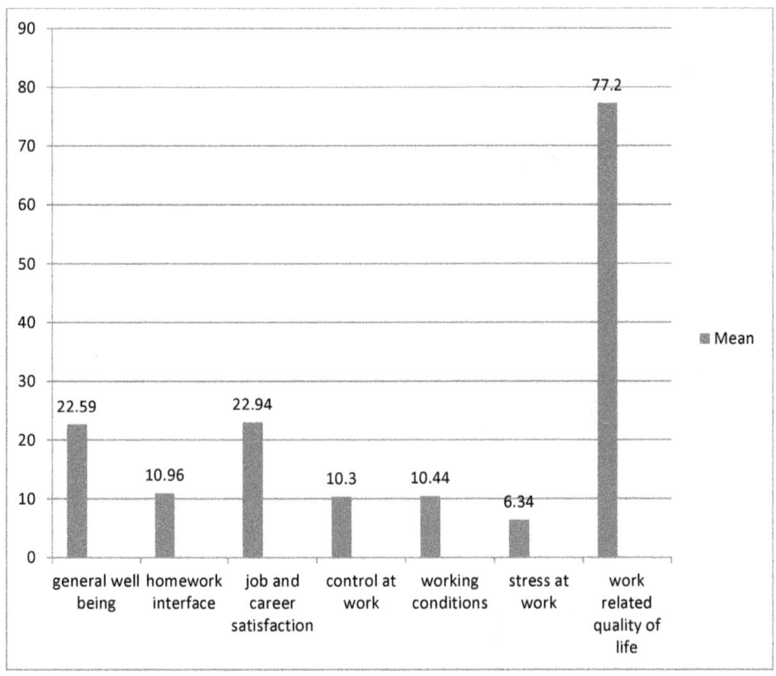

Figure 4.3: Mean's scores for general wellbeing, homework interface, job and career satisfaction, control at work, working conditions, stress at work and work related quality of life are shown (N=300).

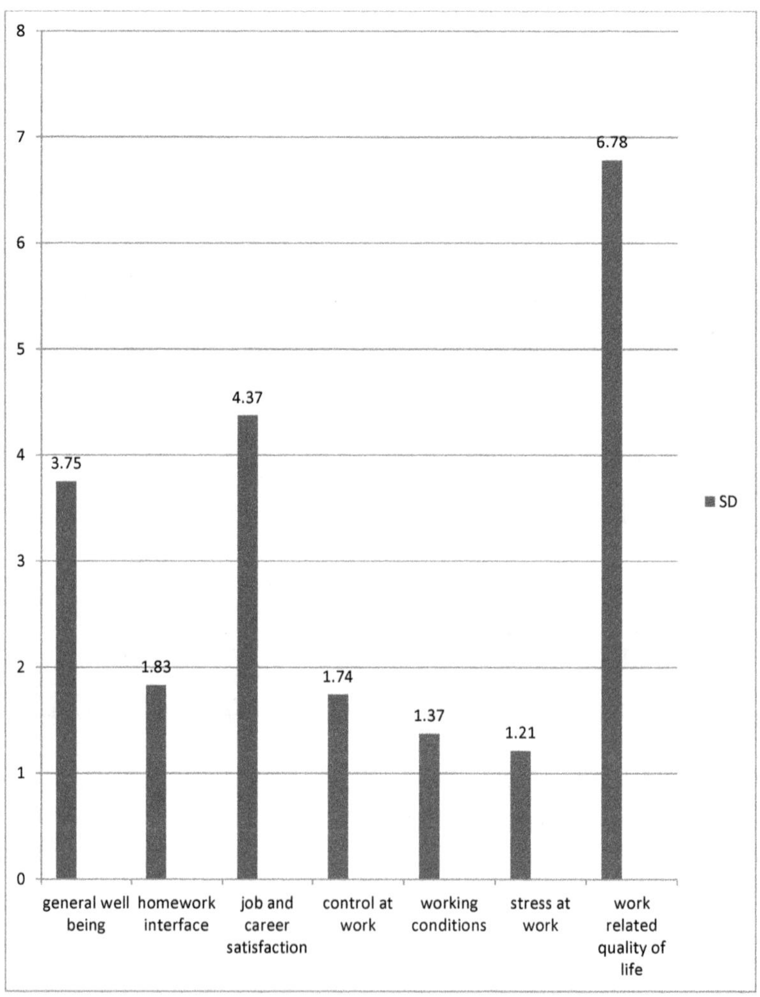

Figure 4.4: SD's scores for general wellbeing, homework interface, job and career satisfaction, control at work, working conditions, stress at work and work related quality of life are shown (N=300).

SECTION-II

(CORRELATIONALANALYSIS)

(Pearson Product moment coefficient of correlation)

This section deals with another statistical technique that is called correlation analysis. This is a bivariate analysis that explains the mutual connection or association between two or more variables. The main result or value of correlation is called correlation coefficient and it is denoted by 'r'. The range of a correlation coefficient is from -1 to+1. The value of 'r' explains the strength and direction of association. A Coefficient value nearer to 0 (either positive or negative) shows little or no correlation or Association between the two constructs. A coefficient valuenearerto+1or-1shows Strong relationship between the two variables.

The objective of the present research is – *"To investigate the relationship between quality of sleep, positive emotions, negative emotions, impulsivity and empathy, general well-being, homework interface, job and career satisfaction, control at work, working conditions, and stress at work- and work-related quality of life."*

Table 4.2: Inter-correlation matrix between quality of sleep, positive emotions, negative emotions, impulsivity, empathy general wellbeing, homework interface, job and career satisfaction, control at work, working conditions, stress at work and work related quality of life among Doctors (N=300).

Variables	1	2	3	4	5	6	7	8	9	10	11	12
Sleep	1	-.844**	.492	.633*	-.868**	-.795**	-.833**	-.837**	-.815**	-.680*	.719*	-.822**
Positive		1	-.470	-.737*	.754*	.963**	.954**	.974**	.978**	.862**	-.930**	.963**
Negative			1	.320	-.497	-.463	-.557	-.444	-.449	-.364	.465	-.459
Impulsivity				1	-.554	-.834**	-.870**	-.819**	-.833**	-.965**	.879**	-.876**
Empathy					1	.786**	.788**	.807**	.772**	.594	-.701*	.770**
Wellbeing						1	.980**	.994**	.996**	.926**	-.986**	.990**
Homework							1	.978**	.984**	.941**	-.973**	.992**
Job								1	.996**	.913**	-.968**	.992**
Control Work									1	.931**	-.980**	.995**
Work condition										1	-.960**	.953**
Stress											1	-.980**
Work Total												1

**Significant at 0.01 level.

Table No. 2 lists the correlation coefficient between quality of sleep, positive emotions, negative emotions, impulsivity, empathy general wellbeing, homework interface, job and career satisfaction, control at work, working conditions, stress at work and work related quality of life among doctors.

Quality of Sleep & Its Correlates

As seen from the above table, a positive relationship was found between poor quality of sleep and impulsivity (r= .633, p< 0.05) and stress (r= .719, p< 0.05) among doctors. A negative association was found between poor quality of sleep and positive emotions (r= -.844, p< 0.01), empathy (r= -.868, p< 0.01) , wellbeing (r= -.795, p< 0.01) , homework interface (r= -.833, p< 0.01), job and career satisfaction (r= -.837, p< 0.01), control at work (r= -.815, p< 0.01), working conditions (r= -.680, p< 0.05) and overall work quality of sleep (r= -.822, p< 0.01) among doctors.

No significant relationship was found between quality of sleep and negative emotions (r= .492, p> 0.05) among doctors. Previous studies support present study Stricker, Brown, Wetherell, and Drummond (2009) present empirical existing research that regions of the brain's prefrontal cortex, which supports mental capabilities such as working memory as well as logical and practical reasoning, showed increased activity in sleepier subjects as they attempted to compensate for the negative effects of poor sleep quality. The effects of the quality of sleep on physicians are underrated. Poor quality of sleep can make an individual unhealthy and can lead to mor negative kind of effects like lacking a good quality sleep, feel less energetic all the time, not able to focus upon their goals and less empathetic behavior. Studies have also shown that irritability increase with poor sleep. Often, people having less sleep in a whole day found to be hallucinating about things and objects.

Positive Emotions & Its Correlates

A positive association was found between positive emotions and empathy (r= .754, p< 0.05), wellbeing (r= .963, p< 0.01), homework interface (r= .954, p< 0.0), job and career satisfaction(r= .974, p< 0.01), control at work (r= .978, p< 0.01) and working conditions (r= .862, p< 0.01) among doctors whereas a negative correlation as found between positive emotions and impulsivity (r= -.737, p< 0.05) and stress (r= -.930, p< 0.01).

No significant relationship was found between positive emotions and negative emotions (r= .470, p> 0.05) among doctors. Cheung and Tang (2009) investigate the links between emotional labour, work family interference, and work quality of life. 442 Chinese service employees in Hong Kong provided self-reported data for a cross-sectional study. Even though the principles of organisational display or demographic data of employees were controlled, the results of correlation with hierarchical regression analysis revealed that surface behaviour has a substantial correlation with work-to-family interference.

Negative Emotions & Its Correlates

No significant relationship was found between positive emotions and other variables taken for study.

Impulsivity & Its Correlates

A positive relationship was found between impulsivity and stress (r= .879, p< 0.05). On the other side, a negative association was seen between impulsivity and wellbeing (r= -.834, p< 0.01), homework interface (r= -.870, p< 0.0), job and career satisfaction (r= -.819, p< 0.01), control at work (r= -.833, p< 0.01), working (r= -.965, p< 0.01) and overall quality of work life (r= -.876, p< 0.01) among doctors.

No significant relationship was found between impulsivity and empathy (r= .554, p> 0.05). study by Al-Masri (2020) showed that there was a link between impulsive purchase behaviour and emotional balance among students from Petra University Accounting Department and Al-Imam Mohammad Ibn Saud Islamic University, based on nationality, gender, and economic status. The study discovered a negative relationship between impulsive purchasing and emotional equilibrium.

Empathy & Its Correlates

A positive association was found between empathy and wellbeing (r= .786, p< 0.01), homework interface (r= .788, p< 0.0), job and career satisfaction (r= .807, p< 0.01), control at work (r= .772, p< 0.01) and overall quality of work life (r= .770, p< 0.01) among doctors. A negative relationship was found between empathy and stress (r= -.701, p< 0.05).

No significant relationship was found between empathy and working conditions (r= .594, p> 0.05). Previous research help in present study Moudatsou's current work (2020) is an integrative but also analytical literature study on the idea and meaning of empathy among health and social care professionals. Health care providers that have a high level of empathy have been demonstrated to be more effective in their function in inducing therapeutic change.

Wellbeing & Its Correlates

A positive correlation was found between wellbeing and homework interface (r= .980, p< 0.0), job and career satisfaction (r= .994, p< 0.01), control at work (r= .996, p< 0.01), working conditions (r= .926, p< 0.01) and overall quality of work life (r= .990, p< 0.01). A negative association was found between wellbeing and stress (r= -.986, p< 0.01).

Homework Interface & Its Correlates

A positive association was found between homework interface and job and career satisfaction (r= .978, p< 0.01), control at work (r= .984, p< 0.01), working conditions (r= .941, p< 0.01) and overall quality of work life (r= .992, p< 0.01) among doctors. A negative correlation was found between homework interface and stress (r= -.973 p< 0.01).

Job and Career Satisfaction & Its Correlates

A positive relationship was found between job and career satisfaction and control at work (r= .996, p< 0.01), working conditions (r= .913, p< 0.01) and overall quality of work life (r= .992, p< 0.01) whereas a negative association was found between job and career satisfaction and stress (r= -.968 p< 0.01) among doctors.

Control at Work & Its Correlates

A positive correlation was found between control at work and working conditions (r= .931, p< 0.01) and overall quality of work life (r= .995, p< 0.01). A negative association was seen between control at work and stress (r= -.980 p< 0.01) among doctors.

Working Conditions & Its Correlates

A significant relationship was seen between working condition and overall quality of work life (r= .953, p< 0.01) and stress (r= -.960 p< 0.01) among doctors.

Stress & Its Correlates

A significant negative relationship was found between stress and overall quality of life (r= -.980 p< 0.01) among doctors.

It can be said from the above table that there has to be open and healthy environment to improve quality of work life. To grow and to flourish at workplace, one needs to be positive towards our colleagues and subordinates. Some of the variables are positively related with quality of work life i.e. positive, empathy, wellbeing, homework interface, job and career satisfaction, positive working conditions and good quality of sleep. When we talk about quality of work life and positive emotions, they are strongly related with each other.

Positive attitude towards workplace and vice versa leads to a better healthy life at workplace as well as at home. If one wants to grow stronger than one had to focus upon happiness and good quality of work life. Emotional and social support from subordinates at workplace can actually make an individual calm and happy. When we talk about work related quality of life and empathy, it literally states that better quality standards at workplace can actually help an individual in understanding other emotions and one tries to feel for their emotions too.

As we are social animal, one had to be empathetic towards others so that we can spread words of joy together. Good quality of work life also leads to better physical, mental and social health. Wellbeing is a state of comfort, happiness and healthy life style which is usually maintained by focusing on good quality work. Good quality of work life also means that when an individual finishes his/her work at workplace only, workers tries not to mix his/ her personal and professional life.

Job satisfaction is directly related with good quality of work life. Technical and social support from co-workers makes a job easy looking and it also increases job satisfaction which is a sub component of career satisfaction. Quality of work life is also been positively related with good quality of sleep. Getting satisfaction on a daily basis from workplace helps in taking a beauty sleep and healthy sleep at night. There has been numerous studies which stated that quality of work life also increases work productivity and its good for long run in life as it helps in boosting our self-confidence.

H2: The second hypothesis suggests *"there would be negative significant relationship between mood swings and work related quality of life."*

The statistically significant variables, their direction and coefficient value with general well-being have been shown in figure 5

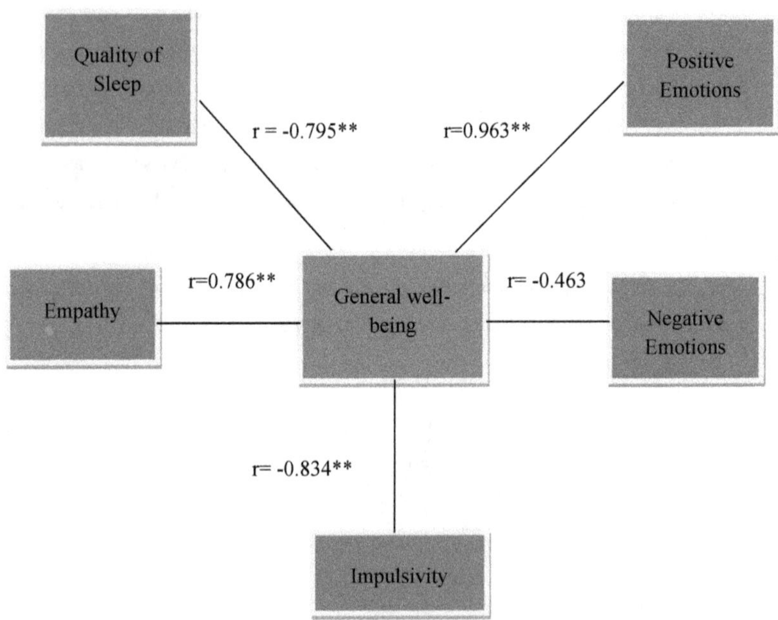

Figure 4.5: *Significant correlates of general well-being.*

The statistically significant variables, their direction and coefficient value with homework interface have been shown in figure 6.

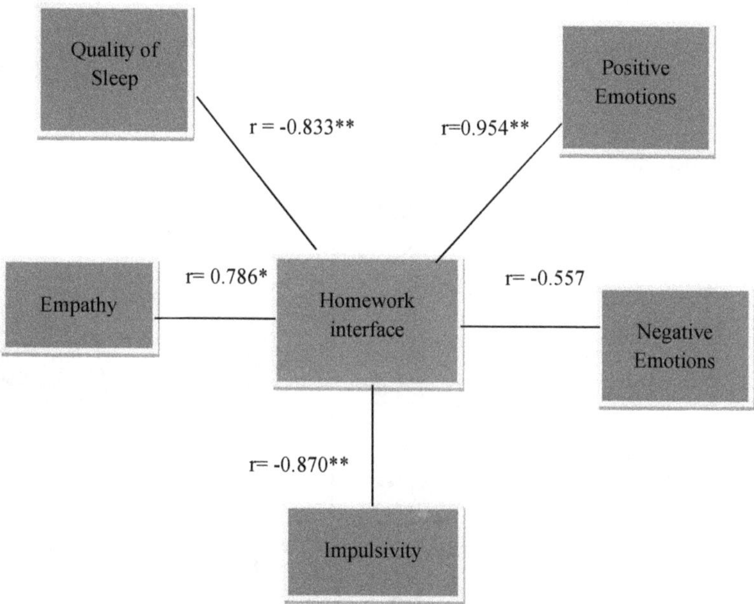

Figure 4.6: Significant correlates of homework interface.

The statistically significant variables, their direction and coefficient value with job and career have been shown in figure 7

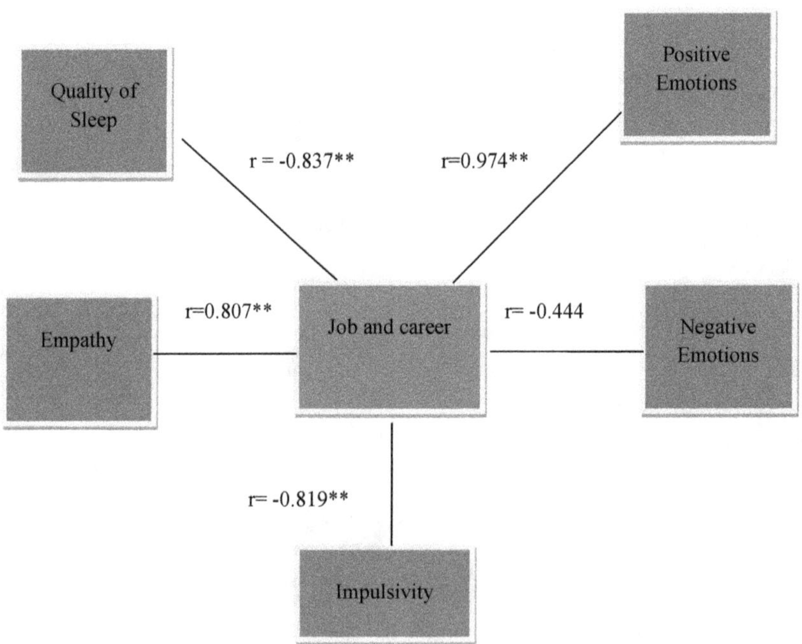

Figure 4.7: Significant correlates of job and career.

The statistically significant variables, their direction and coefficient value with control of work have been shown in figure 8.

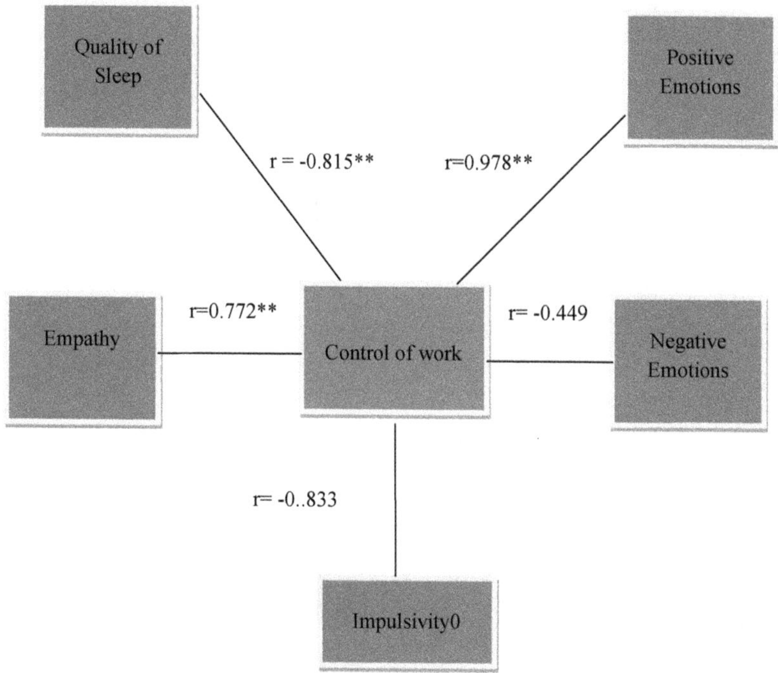

Figure 4.8: Significant correlates of control of work.

The statistically significant variables, their direction and coefficient value with work conditions have been shown in figure 9

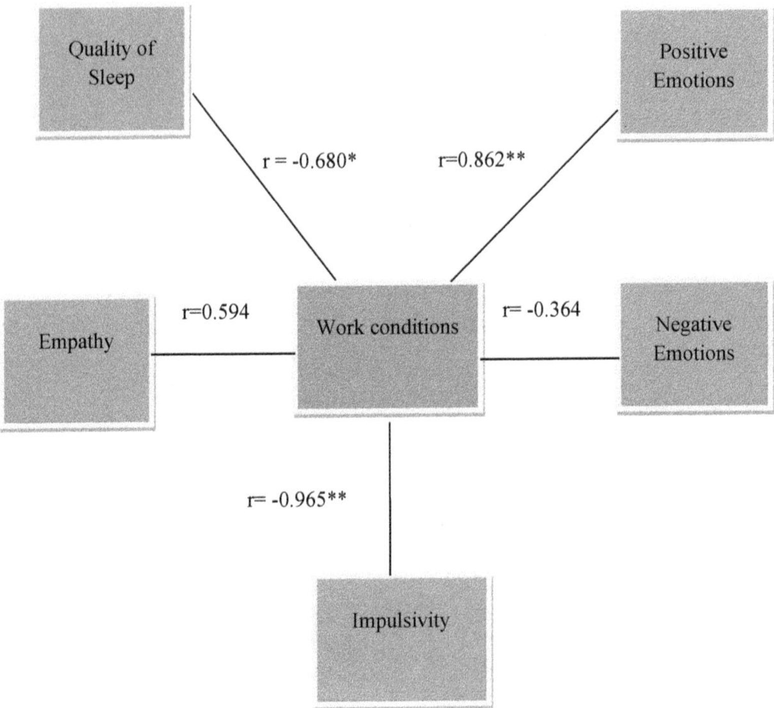

Figure 4.9: *Significant correlates of work conditions.*

The statistically significant variables, their direction and coefficient value with stress on work have been shown in figure 10.

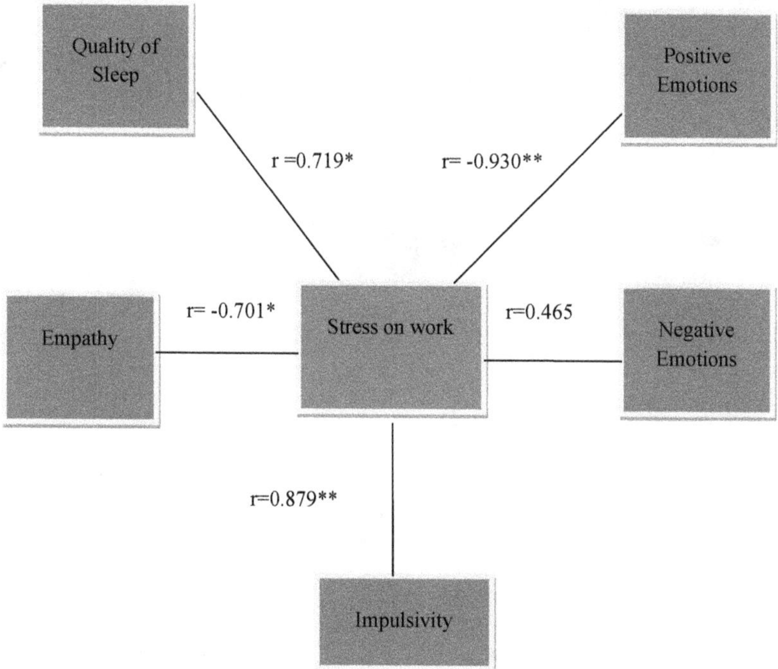

Figure 4.10: *Significant correlates of stress on work.*

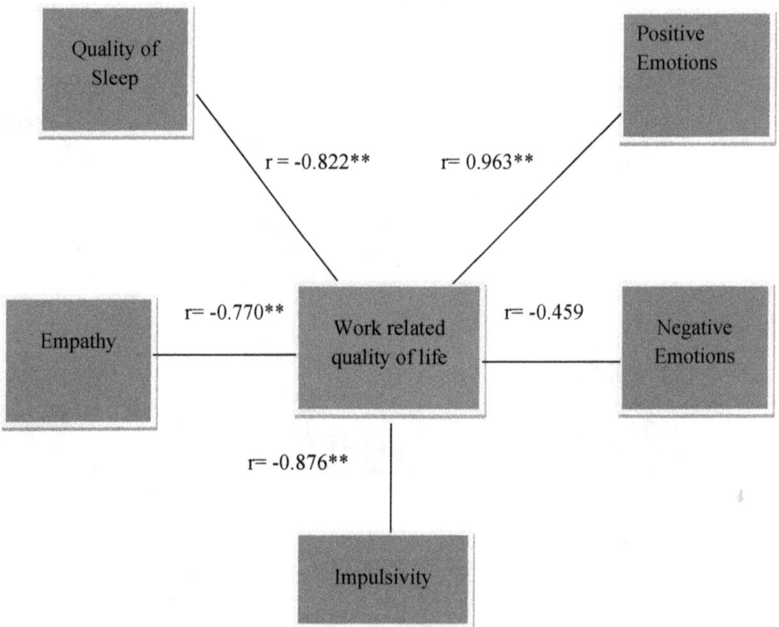

Figure 4.11: Significant correlates of Work Related Quality of Life

SECTION- III

REGRESSION ANALYSIS

(Stepwise Multiple Regression)

The previous section of this chapter talked about correlation analysis and it was found that almost all the variables taken for the present research were significantly related with adolescent aggression. Significant relationship between the variables have provided the base to go further for higher statistics i.e. regression analysis by using stepwise multiple regression method. Regression analysis is *"a set of statistical processes for estimating the relationships between a dependent variable (often called the 'outcome variable') and one or more independent variables (often called 'predictors', 'covariates', or 'features'). Regression analysis is primarily used for two conceptually distinct purposes. First, regression analysis is widely used for prediction and forecasting, where its use has substantial overlap with the field of machine learning.*

Second, in some situations regression analysis can be used to infer causal relationships between the independent and dependent variables. Importantly, regressions by themselves only reveal relationships between a dependent variable and a collection of independent variables in a fixed dataset. To use regressions for prediction or to infer causal relationships, respectively, a researcher must carefully justify why existing relationships have predictive power for a new context or why a relationship between two variables has a causal interpretation". There are mainly two types of regression i.e. linear regression and multiple regression. For the present research, we will be using multiple regression because the independent or predictor variables are more than one in our study. This technique is also called Multiple Regression Analysis.

62

Table 4.3: Stepwise multiple regression analysis for predicting Quality of Work Life from positive emotions, negative emotions, impulsivity, empathy and work related quality of life among Doctors (N=300).

Doctors		
Predictors	**ΔR^2**	**B**
Step 1 Quality of Sleep	.410	.301
Step 2 Positive Emotion	.116	.207
Step 3 Negative Emotion	.023	-.080
Step 4 Impulsivity	.019	-.221
Step 5 Empathy Total R^2	.025 .593	.192
N	300	

It can be observed from the Table 3 that quality of sleep total has been found to be the main positive predictor of doctor's work related quality of life with 41% (β= 0.301) of variance. Positive emotion total also explain positive prediction 11.6% (β= 0.207) of variance respectively with doctor's work related quality of life. 2.3% of the v ariance is significantly predicted by negative emotions total in relation with doctor's work related quality of life with beta value as -0.080. Impulsivity total is the variable among the other variables which is a negative predictor of doctor's work related quality of life with 1.9% with the beta value as -0.221. Empathy total showed a significant predictor of 2.5% (β= 0.192) variance with adolescent aggression

It can be concluded from the study that the quality of sleep total and positive emotions total are highly correlated with adolescent aggression. The predictor variable that has the highest R with the criterion variable, moral disengagement total, is the first variable entered into the analysis. The predictor variable that has the lowest R with the criterion variable, father's hostile aggression, is the last entered variable into the analysis. Thus, stepwise multiple regression helped in finding out the best and suitable predictors of adolescent aggression out of all the variables. Hypothesis is partially accepted.

The major findings are also reported in **figure 12** with the help of pie chart diagram.

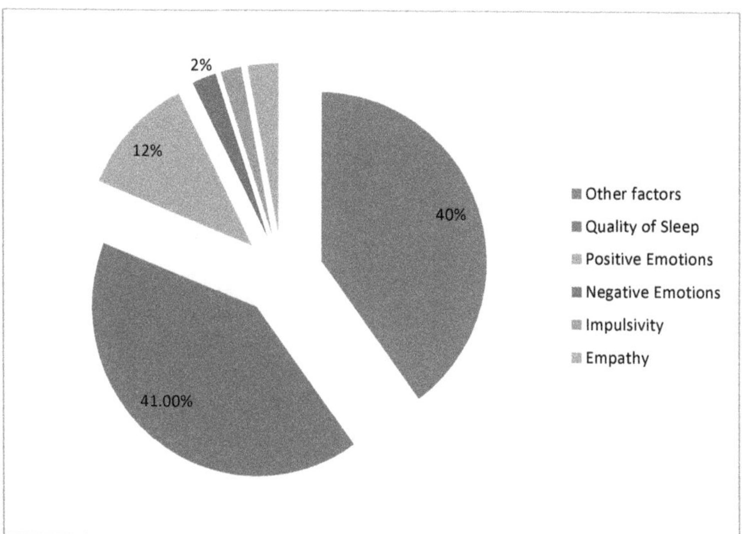

Figure 4.12: Contribution of Quality of Work Life from positive emotions, negative emotions, impulsivity, empathy and work related quality of life among Doctors (N=300).

Graph No. 4.13 Representing the Partial Regression Plot of doctors for the Criterion Variable Work related quality of life and Predictor Variable quality of sleep.

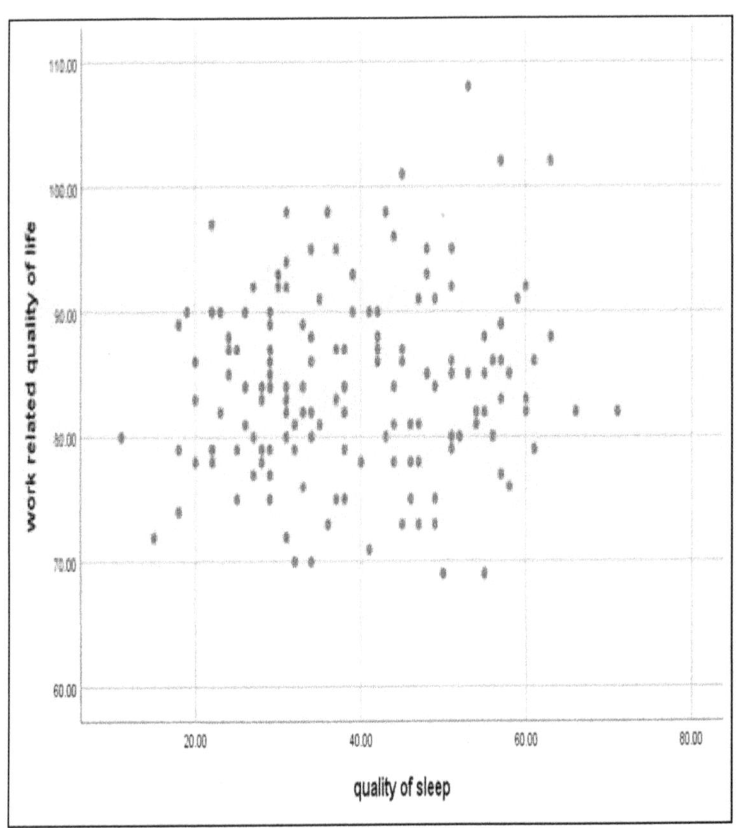

work related quality of life
quality of sleep

Graph No. 4.14   Representing the Partial Regression Plot of doctors for the Criterion Variable Work related quality of life and Predictor Variable positive emotions.

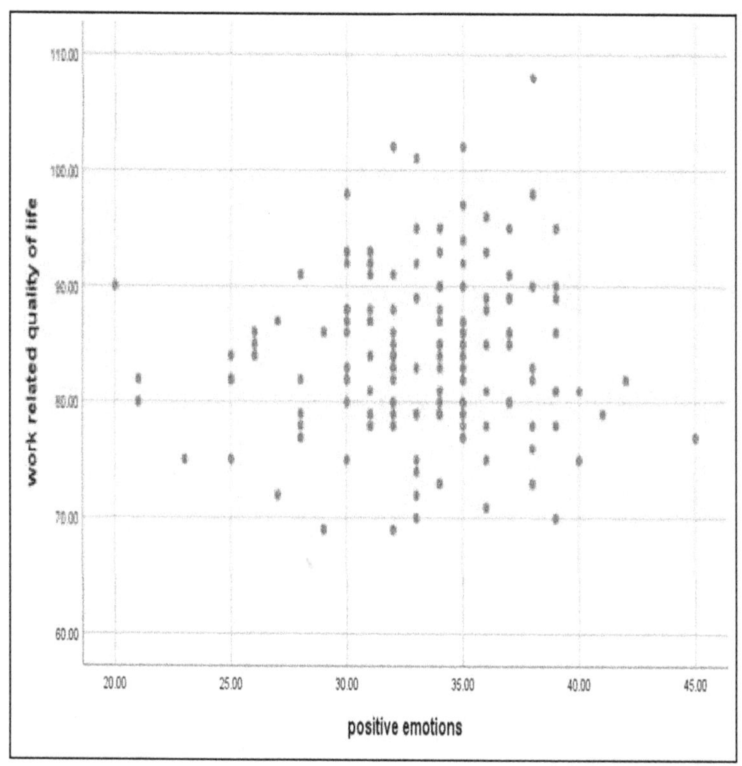
work related quality of life
positive emotions
110.00
100.00
90.00
80.00
70.00
60.00
20.00
25.00
30.00
35.00
40.00
45.00

Graph No. 4.15 Representing the Partial Regression Plot of doctors for the Criterion Variable Work related quality of life and Predictor Variable negative emotions.

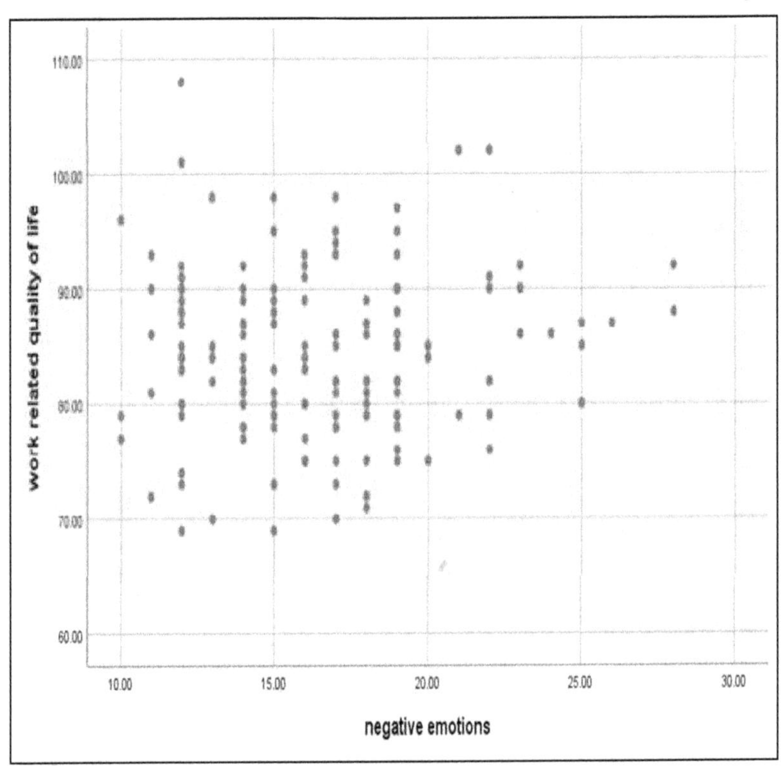
work related quality of life
negative emotions

Graph No. 4.16 Representing the Partial Regression Plot of doctors for the Criterion Variable Work related quality of life and Predictor Variable impulsivity.

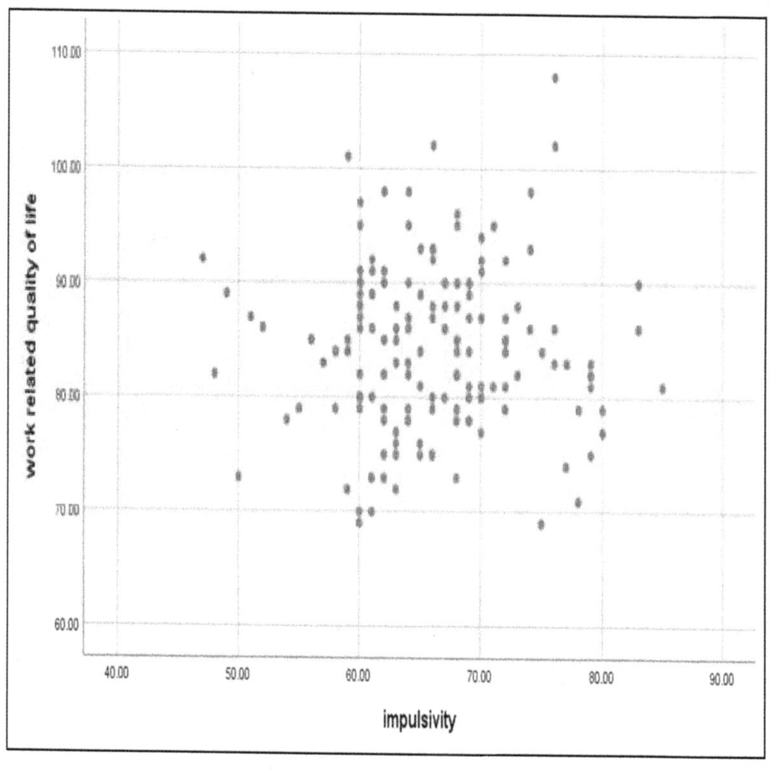
work related quality of life
impulsivity

Graph No. 4.17 Representing the Partial Regression Plot of doctors for the Criterion Variable Work related quality of life and Predictor Variable empathy.

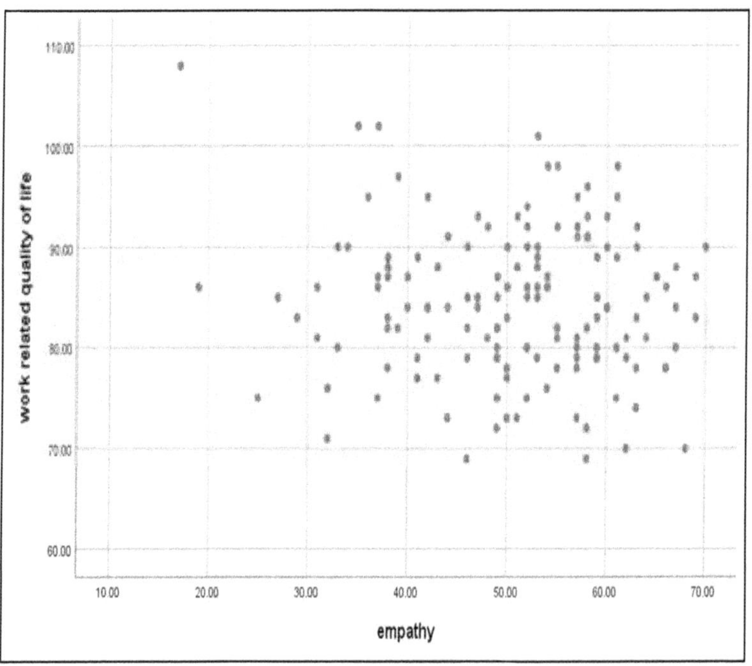

Implications

The aim of the present study was to study quality of sleep, mood swings, impulsivity and empathy in relation to work related quality of life in doctors.

Since the study has been conducted on medical professionals in relation to quality of sleep, mood swings, impulsivity and empathy as independent variables while work related quality of life as dependent or performance variables. Findings reveal that the quality of sleep in medical professionals is partially disturbed. The reason can be attributed to their more hectic and rigorous life style during corona times when pandemic was at its peak. At the same time these doctors have been found more full of positive emotions and empathic with their patients because they have been taken as warriors.

These findings clearly state that human resource is the asset of any organization and the organization needs to cater and enhance the overall willingness of its employees by conducting life skill workshops time to time. Especially during these times when we all are facing adverse and unpredictable scenario of our means of livelihood. This study is very fruitful as it has its behavioral applied value when the need of the hour is to suggest to policy makers and provide conducive environment abstract with positive emotions to their employees so that their employees can be more productive and high output to their work set up. Such type of study can be very helpful in designing some tailor made programs which enhance the work related quality of life in terms of personal effectiveness, efficiency and the well being of employees. Time to time such short term training programs if conducted at different levels would be able to increase the productivity of an organization.

Limitations

o   If the similar kind of study needs to be conducted in future also, then the sample size should be large because it can lead to more effective results.

o   Different organizational sectors or job sectors like government hospitals vs. Private hospitals could have been taken up and also be compared with each other to study some other perspective.

o   More variables should have been used in the present study like happiness, burnout, job satisfaction etc.

o   More demographic variables could have been taken like sex, salary per month, rural- urban background, work load etc.

o   There could have been lack of partial adequacy in data collection as it was done online and in times on Covid – 19.

SUMMARY

Doctors are the most important form of healthcare available to us today. Their daily life requires them to take ultimate responsibility for difficult decisions in situations of clinical complexity and uncertainty, drawing on their scientific knowledge and well developed clinical judgment. Doctors are a specialized subset of healthcare workers and a vital component of frontline health care that often have to cope with a heavy workload in their workplace, sometimes an unhealthy work environment, long working hours or mandatory overtime, and can have high levels of stress. The wellbeing of doctors may relate directly to the quality of patient care. Doctors as clinical scientists apply the principles and procedures of medicine to prevent, diagnose, care for and treat patients with illness, disease and injury and to maintain physical and mental health. They supervise the implementation of care and treatment plans by others in the health care team and conduct medical education and research.

For a healthcare organization to survive, the key resource is a doctor. A doctor's place in the healthcare industry may be regarded as important healthcare gatekeepers and custodians. It can, therefore, be stated that approaching a healthcare organization and deriving benefits directly means consulting a doctor. The healthcare sector increasingly depends on the doctors for their patients. In the 21st century healthcare industry, the life of a doctor is hectic and requires a lot of energy, evidently doctors also get tired and need a peaceful sleep. The kind of sleep a person has the previous night has a lot of impact on the person's mood, freshness, attitude the next day. The need for getting sleep cannot be overemphasized. Lack of sleep quality is related to a number of acute and chronic problems challenging our day to day life. Sleep is a vital part of human physiology and disorders of sleep can result in significant derangement of human functionality.

Now the question is, if a doctor is working late the night before and hasn't had enough sleep, wouldwe want him to perform his duty the next day? These things are completely opposite to the virtuesof a doctor and the ethical moral code they vow to follow, which makes good quality of sleep an important factor in the overall mental and physical health of a doctor.

Quality of sleep

Sleep quality refers to how well you sleep. For adults, good quality sleep means typically falling asleep in 30 minutes or less, sleeping soundly through the night with no more than one awakening, and drifting back to sleep within 20 minutes if we do wake up. The key determinants of quality sleep according to The National Sleep Foundation (2019) are: sleeping more time while in bed (at

least 85 percent of the total time), falling asleep in 30 minutes or less, waking up no more than once per night; and being awake for 20 minutes or less after initially falling asleep.

Lack of good quality sleep can lead to physical and mental health problems, injuries, loss of productivity and even greater risk of death. Quality of sleep can vary due to voluntary behavior, people who engage in voluntary, but unintentional, chronic sleep deprivation are classified as having a sleep disorder called behaviorally induced insufficient sleep syndrome. This is a type of hypersomnia. It involves a pattern of restricted sleep that is present almost daily for at least three months. Other reasons for lack of sleep quality can be long working hours, personal obligations and medical conditions.

Cates, Clark, Woolley and Saunders(2015) believe that sleep is directly related to health and quality of life, is a basic need for a human being to continue his bio-psycho-social and cultural functions. Sleep affects the quality of life and health, which is also perceived as an important variable (Engin & Ozgur, 2004). (Aysan, Karakose, Zaybak & Ismailoglu, 2014) found out that feeling energetic and fit after sleeping is described as the sleep quality. The fact that, nowadays the complaints about sleep disorder being prevalent, low sleep quality being an indicator of many medical diseases and there is strong relationship between physical ,psychological wellness and sleep; sleep quality is an important concept in the clinic practices and related researches on sleep (Keshavarz Akhlaghi & Ghalebandi, 2009)

A sleep restricted state can cause fatigue, daytime sleepiness, clumsiness and increased appetite leading to weight gain (Taheri & Lin, 2004) and it also affects the brain and cognitive functioning (Alhola & Kantola, 2007). For most adults, the amount of sleep needed for best health is seven to eight hours each night. When we get less sleep than that, as many people do, it can eventually leadto a host of health problems. These are forgetfulness, inattentiveness, low immunity, and even mood swings. Quality of sleep is becoming poorer as many people try to adjust their schedule to get as much done as possible, and sleep gets sacrificed. Older adults need as much sleep as the younger adults; they typically sleep more lightly and for shorter time spans than younger people.

Several studies have examined correlations between sleep quality and how the individual feels immediately on waking and during the day.(Argyropoulos, Hicks &Nash, 2003) The results indicate that sleep quality is associated with ease of waking, tiredness, sense of balance and coordination clear-headedness, how rested, restored and refreshed one feels, and mood and physical feelings on waking. During the day, feelings of tiredness predicted poorer sleep quality and alertness predicted better sleep quality.

According to Saygili, Akinci, Arikan and Dereli (2011) sleep quality is affected from the external factors such as gender, academic success, academic background, general health, socio-economic status and the stress level of the person, according to. It has also been found out by Mayda, Kasap, Yildirim, Yilmaz, Derdiyok and Ertan (2012) that medical students may have sleep issues due to their training program being though, time and effort-requiring. Because of this matter, students who cannot sleep enough may have various physical, social, psychological problems.

An empirical research evidence by Stricker, Brown, Wetherell and Drummond (2009) shows that regions of the brain's prefrontal cortex, an area that supports mental faculties such as working memory and logical and practical reasoning, displayed more activity in sleepier subjects as they were trying to compensate for adverse effects caused by poor quality of sleep.

The effects of sleep quality on doctors are underrated. Poor sleep quality can easily lead to lower levels of effort, lower levels of trust, lower levels of empathy and mood swings. Mood swings increase agitation and keep the body aroused, awake and alert which makes it difficult to sleep. Quality of sleep and mood swings is correlated with each other.

Mood Swings

A mood swing is an extreme or rapid change in mood. When mood swings are so strong that they are disruptive, they may be the main part of a bipolar disorder. Mood swings can happen anytime at any place, varying from the microscopic to the wild oscillations of manic depression, so the continuum can be traced from normal struggles around self –esteem, up to a depressive disease

The duration of mood swings also varies. They may last a few hours (ultra rapid) or extend over days (ultrafine). Clinicians maintain that when four continuous days of hypomania, or seven days of mania, occur, is a diagnosis of bipolar disorder justified (Ghaemi,2007).In such cases, mood swings can extend over several days, even weeks: these episodes may consist of rapid alternation between feelings of depression and euphoria (Hockenbury, Don & Sandra, 2011).

Changes in a person's energy level sleep patterns, self-esteem, concentration, drug or alcohol use can be signs of an oncoming mood disorder. Many different things might trigger mood swings, from unhealthy diet or lifestyle to drug abuse or hormonal imbalance. Other major causes of mood swings (besides bi-polar disorder and major depression) include diseases/disorders which interfere with nervous system function. Attention Deficit Hyperactivity Disorder (ADHD), epilepsy, and autism are three such examples.

Sleep quality and mood disorders are closely linked. And it can work both ways – quality of sleep can affect mood, and mood can affect quality of sleep. Studies show people who poor sleep quality report increases in negative moods (anger, frustration, irritability, sadness) and decreases in positive moods. Sleeplessness is often a symptom of mood disorders, such as depression and anxiety. It can also raise the risk of, and even contribute to, developing some mood disorders. Mood can also affect sleep. Anxiety and stress increase agitation and keep the body aroused, awake and alert which makes it difficult to sleep.

Effect of on call related sleep deprivation on physician's mood and alertness was researched by Siraj, Wali and Qutah (2003). The purpose of the study was to determine the effect of acute sleep deprivation due to working long on call shifts on mood and alertness. It was concluded that acute loss due to working long on call shifts significantly decreases daytime alertness and negatively affects the mood state.

To document and analyze the quality and quantity of emergency physicians sleep as a function of day and night shift work, and to compare cognitive and motor performance and mood during day and night shifts a study was conducted in the emergency department of Stanford University MedicalCentre and physician's homes. It was concluded that attending emergency physicians get less sleep and are less effective when performing manual and cognitive tests. Subjects also rated themselves significantly less sleepy, happy and clearer thinking when working day versus night. There was strong cumulative evidence to suggest that both the mood and performance of the resident are adversely affected by the usual moderate loss of sleep.

Studies suggest that impulsivity is consistently elevated during mania (Strakowski, Fleck &Delbello, 2009). People at high risk for mania also endorse experiencing heightened impulsivity when in the throes of strong emotion according to Giovanelli, Hoerger, Gruber and Johnson (2013).Based on these preliminary findings, it was said that individuals diagnosed with bipolar I disorder would show elevations in facets of impulsivity associated with reward and strong emotion, and that these forms of impulsivity would most strongly impair psychosocial functioning within this diagnostic group. Mood swings are found to be significantly related to impulsivity, as the mood swings escalate, impulsive behavior also seems to increase.

Impulsivity

Impulsivity is a tendency to act on whim, displaying behavior characterized by little or no forethought, reflection, or consideration of the consequences (VandenBos, 2007). Impulsive actions and typically "poorly conceived, prematurely expressed, unduly risky, or inappropriate to the situation that often result in undesirable consequences (Daruna&Barnes, 1993),which imperil long term goals and strategies for success (Madden, Gregory, Johonson, Patrick, 2010).Moeller and Barret (2001) believed that impulsivity includes readiness to take immediate and unplanned action as a response to internal and external stimuli, with no regard for their negative consequences for themselves or the others. This definition has several features, which are helpful in research and treatment. Firstly, impulsivity is considered as a potential that itself could be considered as a part of behavioral pattern. Secondly, impulsivity includes an immediate and unplanned action that takes place while there has not been enough chance for evaluating the consequences. According to this feature, impulsivity is distinguished from impaired judgment or compulsive behavior in which planning has already taken place before the action. Thirdly, impulsivity indicates taking action with no regard for its consequence.

Impulsivity is known to be related to both internalizing and externalizing problems. Recent research by Johnson, Tharp, Peckham, Carver and Haase (2017) has demonstrated a relationship between emotion-focused impulsivity that triggers action and externalizing problems such as aggression and substance use. In regards to internalizing problems, another emotion-focused facet of impulsivity has been found to be related to depression and anxiety. Specifically, this facet represents the influence of negative emotions on the individual's view of the world and their automatic thoughts.

Impulsivity is both a facet of personality and a major component of various disorders, including ADHD, substance abuse disorders, bipolar disorder (Henry & Chantal, 2001), antisocial personality disorder and borderline personality disorder. Traits that can lead to impulsive actions are urgency, sensation seeking and low consciousness.

Inadequate sleep has been linked to problematic behaviors, such as poor impulse control and emotion dysregulation (Beebe, 2011). Further support for this link between sleep deprivation and impulsivity comes from studies that have found impaired response inhibition, risky decision- making, and increased risk-seeking all associated with sleep deprivation in adulthood (Frings, 2012). Studies suggest that sleepiness (either produced by prolonged and continual wakefulness, fatigue, or accumulated sleep debt) is associated with impulsivity on some neuropsychological tasks. The more aroused, urgent and impulsive a person is, the empathy is less likely to be there. There is a negative relationship between impulsiveness and empathy.

Empathy

According to Hodges and Myers "Empathy is often defined as understanding another person's experience by imagining oneself in that other person's situation. One understands the other person's experience as if it were being experienced by the self, but without the self actually experiencing it."

Empathy is a building block of morality, an absolute essential element that must exist within a doctor. Being able to feel a patient's emotions helps a physician to deliver more compassionate care and make the patient more comfortable during treatment. Research has indicated that doctor's empathy affected patient's psychological parameters and immunity.

According to Reiss (2017), empathy plays a critical interpersonal and societal role, enabling sharing of experiences, needs, and desires between individuals and providing an emotional bridge that promotes pro-social behavior. But studies show empathy declines during medical training. Without targeted interventions, uncompassionate care and treatment devoid of empathy, results in patients who are dissatisfied. They are then much less likely to follow through with treatment recommendations, resulting in poorer health outcomes and damaged trust in health providers. Cognitive empathy must play a role when a lack of emotional empathy exists because of racial, ethnic, religious, or physical differences. Healthcare settings are no exception to conscious and unconscious biases, and there is no place for discrimination or unequal care afforded to patients who differ from the majority culture or the majority culture of healthcare providers. Much work lies ahead to make healthcare equitable for givers and receivers of healthcare from all cultures. Self- and other-empathy leads to replenishment and renewal of a vital human capacity. If we are to move in the direction of a more empathic society and a more compassionate world, it is clear that working to enhance our native capacities to empathize is critical to strengthening individual, community, national, and international bonds.

Martin Hoffman, a psychologist who has worked a lot in the development of empathy, states that everyone is born with the capability of feeling empathy. Human empathy also involves the capacity to take on the perspective of the other. This shift in perspective requires activation of executive control functions in the prefrontal cortex that allows the observer to maintain separate perspectives (Decety&Lamm, 2006).

Emotions motivate individual behavior that aids in solving communal challenges as well as guiding group decisions about societal goodness. Recent research show that individuals who report regular experiences of gratitude exchange are far more likely to help others than those not experiencing a positive emotional state (Bartlett, Desteno 2006). Thus, empathy's influence extends beyond relating to other's emotions, it correlates with an increased positive state and likeliness to aid others.

Empathy is consistently considered an important factor in the development and maintenance of effective therapeutic relationships (Cozolino, 2006; Hubble, Duncan, & Miller, 1999; Lambert & Barley, 2002) as well as an element essential to treatment effectiveness (Greenberg, Elliot, Watson &Bohart, 2001). According to Applegate and Shapiro (2005), it is the therapist's empathy that helps clients to develop the ability to tolerate and regulate their own strong affect, which is a skill that is core to all forms of clinical intervention.

Clinical empathy is an essential element of quality care and is associated with improved patient satisfaction, adherence to treatment, and fewer malpractice complaints. According to Halpern (2012), empathy in medicine is challenging though, because doctors are dealing with the most emotionally distressing situations–illness, dying, suffering in every form–and such situations would normally make an empathic person anxious, perhaps too anxious to be helpful. It is possible that doctors who are most vulnerable to compassion fatigue and emotional distress may fall prey to emotional exhaustion, detachment, and a low sense of accomplishment but the ability to engage in self-other awareness and to regulate one's emotions is pivotal to the adaptive experience of empathy in clinical practice. As the medical profession is struggling to achieve an appropriate balance between work related life satisfaction and empathic concern, these issues require further investigation.

Work related quality of life

Work related quality of life refers to the favorableness or unfavourableness of a job environment for the people working in an organisation. The period of scientific management which focused solely on specialisation and efficiency, has undergone a revolutionary change. The traditional management (like scientific management) gave inadequate attention to human values. In the present scenario, needs and aspirations of the employees are changing. Employers are now redesigning jobs for better QWL.

One of the earliest uses of the term "QoWL" is found in the work of Mayo (1960), but the subsequent 50 years or so has not led to a clear consensus as to how precisely the term should be defined. Many writers have proposed models of QoWL, drawing upon various combinations of factors, based mostly on the orisation, and more rarely on empirical research. Thus Hackman and Oldham (1974) suggested that an individual's psychological growth needs should be addressed in any worthwhile endeavour to increase QoWL. Among the needs they identified were: task identity and significance, autonomy and feedback. Taylor, Cooper, and Mumford (1979) identified other facets of QoWL as key, including what they saw as extrinsic factors such as wages, hours and working conditions, and intrinsic factors associated with the nature of the work itself.

Quality of Working Life (QoWL) as a theoretical concept aims to capture the essence of an individual's work experience in the broadest sense. The QoWL of an individual is influenced by their direct experience of work and by the direct and indirect factors that affect this experience, such as job satisfaction and other factors that broadly reflect life satisfaction and general feeling of well- being (Danna & Griffin, 1999). Improvements to perceived quality of working life have been associated with a range of benefits. For example, the UK's Somerset County Council conducted a study to improve the QoWL of their employees in an attempt to reduce workplace stress and the level of sickness absence within the organization (Tasho, Jordan & Robertson, 2005). It was calculated that the resulting reduction in sickness absence levels from staff (from 10.75 days in 2001-02 to 7.2 days in 2004-05) represented a total net saving of approximately £1.57 million over two years.

One of the many professions that is continuously exposed to prolonged periods of sleep deprivation is that of a resident doctor. In a study by Pikovsky, Oron, Shiyovich, Perr and Nesher (2013) it was found out that the prolonged working hours of resident physicians make them vulnerable to the consequences of sleep penury, which affects their task performance and quality of work life.

Work-Related Quality of Life among Medical Residents at a University Hospital in Northeastern Thailand was researched by Somsila, Chaiear, Boonjaraspinyo and Timkhao (2015). The seven sub-factors were rated as moderate to high for employee engagement and control at work, moderate for home/work interface, general well-being and working conditions, high-moderate for job career satisfaction, and low-moderate for stress at work. The trend showed that working less than eight shifts/ month and working less than 80 hours/week had the potential association with good quality ofwork-life (QWL). It was concluded that the residents and institutions should be better managed to have the appropriate number of working hours and to increase work-life balance, working condition, general well-being, and job-career satisfaction. On the other hand, stress at work must be reduced.

Objectives

- To investigate the relationship between quality of sleep and work related quality of life among doctors.
- To investigate the relationship between mood swings and work related quality of life among doctors.
- To investigate the relationship between impulsivity and work related quality of life among doctors.
- To investigate the relationship between empathy and work related quality of life among doctors.
- To investigate the role of quality of sleep on work related quality of life among doctors.
- To investigate the role of mood swings on work related quality of life among doctors.

- To investigate the role of impulsivity on work related quality of life among doctors.
- To investigate the role of empathy on work related quality of life among doctors.

Hypotheses

- There would be positive relationship between quality of sleep and work relatedquality of life.
- There would be negative relationship between mood swings and work relatedquality of life.
- There would be a negative relationship between impulsivity and work relatedquality of life.
- There would be a positive relationship between empathy and work related quality of life.
- Quality of sleep would act as a significant contributor in Work related quality oflife.
- Mood swings would act as a significant contributor in Work related quality oflife.
- Impulsivity would act as a significant contributor in Work related quality of life.
- Empathy would act as a significant contributor in Work related quality of life.

Research Design:

Fort any type of research, research design works as the backbone. It outlines how the research will be conducted, how it will guide and directs data collection, analysis of data and data reporting. For the present research a correlational design was used.

Sample:

The total sample for the present study was 300 resident doctors. The age of doctors were between 30-35 years, work experience of at least 5 years. The sample was selected from North India region, specifically Haryana, Punjab and NCR region.

Tools used

The following standardized instruments were used for present investigation:

- Sleep Quality Scale
- Positive and Negative Affect schedule (PANAS)
- Barratt Impulsiveness Scale
- Empathy Quotient
- The Work related Quality of Life scale

Implications

The aim of the present study was to study quality of sleep, mood swings, impulsivity and empathy in relation to work related quality of life in doctors.

Since the study has been conducted on medical professionals in relation to quality of sleep, mood swings, impulsivity and empathy as independent variables while work related quality of life as dependent or performance variables. Findings reveal that the quality of sleep in medical professionals is partially disturbed. The reason can be attributed to their more hectic and rigorous life style during corona times when pandemic was at its peak. At the same time these doctors have been found more full of positive emotions and empathic with their patients because they have been taken as warriors.

These findings clearly state that human resource is the asset of any organization and the organization needs to cater and enhance the overall willingness of its employees by conducting life skill workshops time to time. Especially during these times when we all are facing adverse and unpredictable scenario of our means of livelihood. This study is very fruitful as it has its behavioral applied value when the need of the hour is to suggest to policy makers and provide conducive environment abstract with positive emotions to their employees so that their employees can be more productive and high output to their work set up. Such type of study can be very helpful in designing some tailor made programs which enhance the work related quality of life in terms of personal effectiveness, efficiency and the well being of employees. Time to time such short term training programs if conducted at different levels would be able to increase the productivity of an organization.

Limitations

- o If the similar kind of study needs to be conducted in future also, then the sample size should be large because it can lead to more effective results.
- o Different organizational sectors or job sectors like government hospitals vs. Private hospitals could have been taken up and also be compared with each other to study some other perspective.
- o More variables should have been used in the present study like happiness, burnout, job satisfaction etc.
- o More demographic variables could have been taken like sex, salary per month, rural- urban background, work load etc.
- o There could have been lack of partial adequacy in data collection as it was done online and in times on Covid – 19.

CPSIA information can be obtained
at www.ICGtesting.com
Printed in the USA
BVHW091513020123
655321BV00013B/923